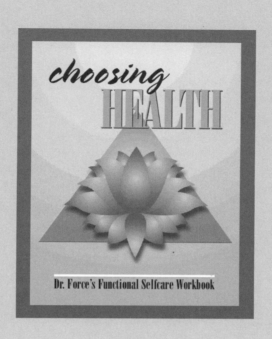

choosing HEALTH
Dr. Force's Functional Selfcare Workbook

The Elements of Health
7500 E. Pinnacle Peak Rd., Suite A-207
Scottsdale AZ 85255
Phone: 480-563-4256
Toll-free: 866-563-4256
Fax: 480-563-4269
Email: info@theelementsofhealth.com
Web: theelementsofhealth.com

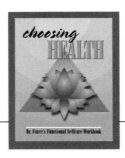

choosing HEALTH

For **permission to reprint** pages from this workbook for educational purposes or to order additional **workbooks**, contact:

The Elements of Health
480-563-4256
866-563-4256 toll-free

or visit our website at:
theelementsofhealth.com

ISBN 0-9723008-0-5

This workbook is not for the treatment or cure of any disease. It is for the purpose of identifying body function and understanding what can be done to support body function. It is based on the principles of functional medicine—restoring health by restoring function. It does not replace the role of a physician.

This workbook is intended to empower you to know how your body functions, what you need to do to function better, be able to measure the results of your work, and know when it is in your best interest to seek further help from a physician who is trained and licensed to diagnose.

The recommendations made in this workbook with regard to the use of products from Biotics Research Corporation, Research Nutrition, Dragon River, Kal, Amazon Herb Company, and Yerba Prima are mine alone and may not agree with recommended uses by these companies. This workbook is not intended to replace common sense; you are always responsible for making for your own healthcare decisions.

This workbook is intended for you to be able to make better-informed decisions regarding your health. It is left to your discretion and is solely your responsibility to determine whether these or any other approaches are appropriate for you.

Innumerable thanks to:

George Goodheart – Creator of Applied Kinesiology; in my opinion, the highest expression of Functional Medicine that exists in the world today. He is a brilliant mind, a noble heart, and a gifted physician.

Lance West – He was my model, mentor, and friend. With loving persistence he opened my hands and my heart to the art of healing.

Harry Eidenier – He is the *master alchemist* of human biochemistry, diagnosis, and clinical nutrition. As his apprentice for almost 20 years, I have never ceased to be moved by his knowledge and desire to serve, and am thankful to call him my friend.

Dr. Force's Functional Selfcare Workbook

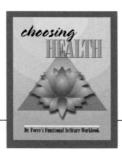

What If...

You were able to know, in a just few minutes, exactly how each part of your body functioned.

You also knew precisely what to do to restore its functions.

You suddenly had answers to health problems that had plagued you for a long time.

You could retest your body systems to determine if whatever you were doing was, indeed, working for you.

You could do this whenever you wanted and it would cost you nothing.

You could read your lab work and know exactly what it all meant.

You could clearly see trends toward illness on your lab work (often, even when your doctor may tell you the findings are perfectly normal) and know precisely what to do to prevent illness before it ever develops.

You knew exactly what elements make for optimum health — and you also knew how to incorporate them into your life so that your life would continually become richer and more rewarding.

You have the tool that will help you do all these things — and much more — **right in your hands!**

This workbook might seem intimidating; it's pretty big. However, the strategies for restoring, optimizing, and protecting your health are easily understood and straightforward.

Think of it as an encyclopedia — an encyclopedia humanica — where you can find answers to questions about your health.

You don't have to read the book cover to cover. Make use of all of the tools and strategies offered in this workbook — or just the ones that work best for you.

Many times over the past thirty years I have been asked to write endorsements and/or critiques for books written by health care providers. Generally, I have complied with the author's wishes.

However, none have been easier than this one. Why? Because in my thirty years in the health care business, I can honestly say I have never had a friend or associate who cared more about getting their patients well.

Dr. Force is an extremely intelligent physician who not only knows what tools to use to help his patients resolve their problem(s), but also more importantly knows how to communicate with them and motivate them to want to help themselves achieve a higher level of health. This is evident throughout this book.

There is a health crisis in this country. Insurance companies (mainly through HMO/PPO plans) now control the health care available to you in this country. Decisions are often made concerning your health on the basis of profitability rather than your needs. In that insurance companies understandably tend to not want to pay until they have to, with disease-prevention health care becoming the exception rather than the norm. The tendency is to pay for heart bypass surgery, for instance, rather than to prevent the heart disease in the first place.

There are more doctors in this country who practice as specialists than there are general and family practitioners. Although specialists are important in health care, it brings to mind the blind men all feeling a different part of an elephant and all believing an elephant is like the leg or the trunk or the tail. They don't see the whole elephant, and thus miss the bigger picture. Modern medicine is often like that, looking ever more closely at smaller and smaller parts and forgetting to see the patient as a whole person.

There now is a need, more than ever, for you to have control over your own health. Though modern medicine can be great when you're in the grips of a health crisis, it's better to avoid the crisis altogether by protecting your health yourself with the tools here.

This workbook is the absolute best guide to self health care I have reviewed. Read it and reread it until you fully understand it, and then begin your journey to better health. Believe me, you will never find a better or more understandable guide. In short, this is the finest book of its type I have ever had the privilege of reviewing.

Harry Eidenier
December 2002

This workbook comes from my twenty years practicing the healing arts. Originally, I was looking for answers for myself; later I was looking for answers for others. I found both in abundance.

Now, I see miracles every day in my practice. People reclaim their lives, overcome illness, become free from pain, regain energy, strength, and mental clarity, and again enjoy the health and well-being that is their birthright.

As wonderful as it is to work with my patients, I can contact only so many people each day. I came to realize that many of the methods and tools I use with my patients could be taught, and that these methods and tools could empower and change the lives of an unlimited number of people. Hence, this workbook was written.

It's a workbook — because it's something you use rather than read. What you have in your hands is a tool that gives you the ability to restore and protect your health.

This is the one and only workbook that teaches you a process called Functional Selfcare. This revolutionary process puts the tools of Functional Medicine (a process in health care that in the past has only been available to physicians) into your hands.

Beyond treating symptoms, this workbook will teach you how to restore health by restoring function.

By using the strategies in this workbook, you will use your symptoms as guides, do home testing, and read your own lab work. You will know exactly where you are, precisely what to do to restore your body functions, and measure the results of your work.

Symptoms and illnesses won't be an elusive mystery anymore; you will have control over your own health.

Mark Force, D.C.
December 2002

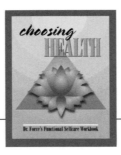

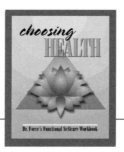

Table of Contents

Table of Contents (Continued)

Choosing Health

A perfection of means and confusion of aims seems to be our main problem. ~ Albert Einstein

The Strategies for Choosing Health

- Realize that most diseases are the result of lifestyle choices.
- Gain the knowledge you need to make effective choices.
- Use functional selfcare to restore and protect your health.
- Keep your doctor on your team.

Realize Most Diseases are the Result of Lifestyle Choices

Most of the diseases people experience are *diseases of choice*. What that means is that most diseases are caused by our habits. There is always a reason why things occur. Disease doesn't just happen; there is always a cause. Most diseases aren't caused by injury — they are caused by the way people live. People's habits — the way they live — either cause disease or prevent disease.

Heart disease, diabetes, cancer, osteoporosis, depression, arthritis, chronic fatigue, menstrual problems, headaches, etc. are most often caused by bad diet, too much stress, not enough exercise, not enough rest, toxic agents (including carcinogens) in your environment, etc.

Most people suffer poor health because they don't know how to make better choices for themselves. Using this workbook, you'll know how to make choices that work for you.

Gain the Knowledge You Need to Make Effective Choices

When you have knowledge, when you know which factors cause disease and which factors cause health, you will have the power of choosing health. You will have the power to prevent most diseases. You will have the power to age with vitality and strength. Once you have knowledge, you have power, because you have conscious choice.

I want you to know what will make you ill and what will make you well. I never want you to be among those who choose disease by default just because you don't know the results of your habits. I want you to be able to choose health.

Use Functional Selfcare to Restore and Protect Your Health

Using functional selfcare is about knowing how your body functions and how to support it to allow optimal functioning and self-healing. Functional selfcare is about taking responsibility for your health day-by-day, week-by-week, and year-by-year.

There are two major aspects of functional selfcare: **The Elements of Health** and **Self-Directed Functional Selfcare**.

The Elements of Health are those strategies everyone needs to use to support their health, such as eating whole and unrefined foods, drinking enough water, and getting adequate sleep and regular exercise.

Self-Directed Functional Selfcare allows you to establish exactly where you are and precisely what to do about your health. When you use the Health Graph, Home Tests, and read your own lab work, the primary tools of self-directed functional selfcare, you will learn the particular needs which must be met for your body to heal.

Keep Your Doctor on Your Team

You still need your doctor! Your doctor plays a critical role in identifying the presence of disease, treating you as needed, and making appropriate referrals based on your needs. Your doctor's remarkable training and expertise allows him or her to give you guidance and help you maintain your health.

Get a yearly physical and listen to your doctor. Take in the information he or she gives you, weigh it out, and make appropriate choices for yourself.

Realms of Functional and Traditional Medicine in the Continuum of Health

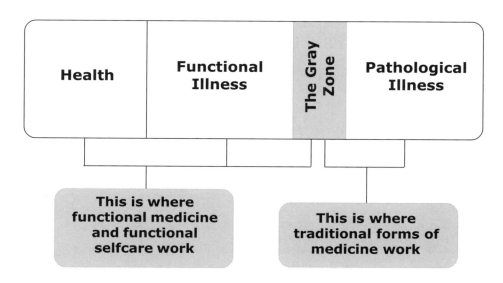

The doctor of the future will give no medicine, but will interest his patient in the care of the (human) frame, in diet and in the cause and prevention of disease. ~ Thomas Edison

Functional Medicine: The Basis for Functional Selfcare

A physician or practitioner of Functional Medicine examines your body to determine how to restore optimal function. Restoring function restores the inherent capacity of your body to heal and regulate itself (homeostasis). Your body cannot heal and regulate itself — cannot keep you healthy — unless its various systems function.

The Principles of Functional Medicine

- Restore health by restoring function.
- Focus on systems and functions.
- Realize that ealth exists as a dynamic continuum.
- See most illnesses as a problem of function.
- Balance all sides of the triad of health: structural, chemical, and mental/emotional.
- Blend the healing arts into a unified approach.
- Use standards based on healthy populations of people.
- Treat healing as an active process.
- Produce measurable results.
- Recognize that individuals and environments are interdependent.
- Use a global and long-term view for your health.

Restore Health by Restoring Function

The inherent capacity of your body to heal and regulate itself is present when your body functions fully. Treating only to control symptoms or manifestations of an illness does not eliminate the cause of an illness. To get well and stay well, you must also treat the cause by determining how your body, mind, and spirit function and what must be done to create the conditions required for optimal function to be present.

Focus on Systems and Functions

Functional Medicine, a systems analysis approach to health care, is a logical and systematic method for evaluating and restoring function to all of your body's systems. Functional Medicine isn't oriented toward solving symptoms or illnesses; rather, the focus is on discovering the cause of a problem and eliminating that cause to restore health.

Treating symptoms rarely restores health. Like painting over rust, you may get an immediate change that looks good, but the rust is still there and always ends up popping through the paint. To be healthy, you have to find all the rust and take everything down to bare metal and then build up from there.

With Functional Medicine, you are more than a collection of parts. You are the summation and mystery that exists beyond the individual tissues, organs, and functions you encompass.

Health Exists as a Dynamic Continuum

Your health is actually a continuum from being perfectly healthy to having fatal illness. You usually don't go straight from being healthy to having a disease. There's a lot of space in between where you may not have a disease, but you aren't healthy either.

Many doctors are trained in a kind of rigid healthy-or-disease way of thinking. That's also the way most diagnostic tests, lab normals, etc. are designed. According to this model, you're either healthy or you have disease. This means many people with functional health problems don't get help because their tests don't show pathological illness.

The Continuum of Health Model and Progression of Illness And Healing

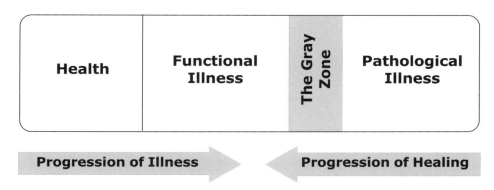

By being able to recognize where you are in the continuum of health, you have leverage to do something about it. The amazing thing is that once you know how to look at a health problem from a functional selfcare perspective, the answers quickly appear. Once you start thinking in terms of how your body works and what you need to do to get it to work for you, a lot of health problems aren't such mysteries anymore.

Most Illnesses are a Problem of Function

Usually illnesses are due to dysfunction rather than pathology (disease). Functional illness causes an unlimited array of symptoms. Virtually any symptom associated with pathological illness or disease can be caused by functional illness. Though essentially any symptom is possible, some of the more common symptoms are headache, joint and muscle pains, insomnia, anxiety, depression, intestinal problems, and chronic fatigue.

The tools of traditional medicine tend to be much more effective for diagnosing and treating pathological illnesses than functional illnesses. Standard interpretation of diagnostic tests and exams often miss functional illnesses. This leaves you vulnerable to the tendency of functional illness developing into disease over time.

Diagnosis and treatment at the functional stage are non-invasive, less costly, and pose fewer risks to your health than diagnosis and treatment of pathological illness. By preventing the development of functional illness, a higher quality of life is maintained throughout life.

Functional Illness: Defining Aspects

- Functional illness is defined as a state where parts of the body are altered in function.
- Functionally altered tissues cannot be separated from those that are healthy.
- The physical structure of the functionally compromised tissues is normal.
- There are rarely medically recognized names for functional illnesses.
- Functional illness represents a very early stage of disease.
- The changes found in functional illness are reversible.

Balance All Sides of the Triad of Health

Functional medicine looks at the totality of who you are and who you are capable of being. Functional medicine looks at who you are genetically, in terms of your inherent strengths and weaknesses, and works toward protecting your health based on that knowledge. Tailoring healthcare specifically to your genetic constitution also supports the fullest expression of your genetic potential. Functional medicine is more than preventing disease; it's about the full expression of your optimal health.

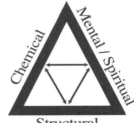

Any of the healing arts can utilize a functional medicine approach, though many disciplines within the healings arts will tend to have unique strengths (and weaknesses) in terms of how broadly and deeply they affect the structural, chemical, and mental aspects of a person's health.

The table on the following page distinguishes the healing arts by their contribution to each aspect of the Triad of Health. Every healing art can include the Triad of Health model. Each healing art is categorized by its most prominent characteristic, but there is overlap. In reality, there is no separation between structure (body and nervous system), chemistry, and mental (mind and spirit). They all are one.

Functional Medicine in the Healing Arts

Structure & Nervous System	Chemical (Body Chemistry)	Mental (Mind and Spirit)
• Acupuncture	• Allopathic Medicine	• Jungian Analysis
• Applied Kinesiology (AK)	• Naturopathic Medicine	• Hypnotherapy
• Chiropractic	• Herbal Medicine	• Neuroemotional Technique
• Massage Therapy	• Homeopathy	• Gestalt Therapy
• Physical Therapy	• Chinese Herbal Medicine	• Transactional Analysis
• Yoga, Tai Chi & Chi Gung	• Ayurvedic Medicine	• Art Therapy
• Weight Training	• Clinical Nutrition	• Music Therapy
• Aerobic Training	• Clinical Ecology	• Breathwork
• Feldenkrais, Pilates and Dance	• Ecological Medicine	• Neurolinguistic Programming
• Osteopathic Medicine	• Orthomolecular Medicine	• Bioenergetics Therapy
• Craniosacral Therapy	• Applied Kinesiology (AK)	• Meditation and Prayer

Blend the Healing Arts into a Unified Approach

Functional Medicine has no hierarchy, either between practitioners of the healing arts or between the practitioners and the individual seeking healing. Whatever the healing art or blending of healing arts that is used for each individual's healing, the sole criteria must be what best serves the healing process. In designing a healing approach, Functional Medicine includes consideration for the individual's goals, beliefs, and aspirations.

Use Standards Based on Healthy Populations

Measuring the health of average groups of people isn't a good enough standard for figuring out how your body functions. The way standard norms are designed for laboratory findings, blood pressures, body temperature, and other physical findings is to test large groups of people at random and to arbitrarily consider that 90% of the people tested are normal (healthy). The 5% at the top end and the 5% at the bottom end are considered abnormal. Having practiced functional medicine for a long time, I can assure you that 90% of people are not healthy.

On the following page are two bell curves. The first bell curve is graphed from the results found for blood glucose (sugar) in an average group of people. This is the standard way that lab normals are determined, and the range for this group is 70 to 110 (this range will vary slightly from lab to lab). The second bell curve is graphed from results found for blood glucose in a healthy group of people. Here the range is 80 to 95 and represents the Optimal Normal Range for glucose.

Standard Medicine Bell Curve for Blood Glucose

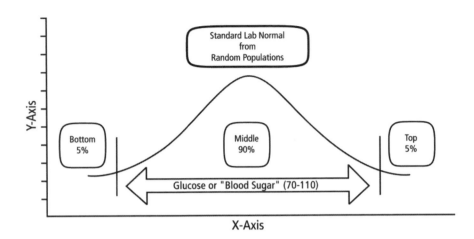

If you test a **healthy** group or population, the bell curve looks different than the one for a general population:

Functional Medicine Bell Curve for Blood Glucose

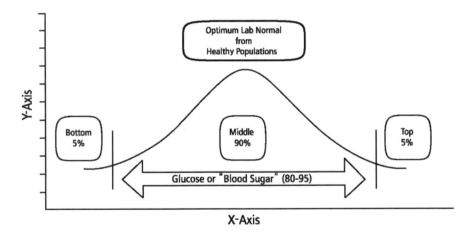

Now you have a parameter for glucose that will tell you if you're actually healthy or not because you're now comparing yourself to a healthy group of people and not an average group of people. If you really want to be healthy, that's the standard you want to use. Believe me, you don't want to use the average group of people because the average person isn't that healthy.

The optimal normal for glucose is an example of the way optimal normal can be figured for any test: use test results from a healthy group to determine what healthy is for that test. Healthy subjects are chosen through patient history and physical exam.

Health Requires Self-Responsibility

It is vitally important for you to know that you are the source of your own healing.

Traditionally, medicine was a passive process; you went to a doctor and the doctor fixed you. This is an appropriate strategy for some health problems. For instance, if you needed surgery, it would be best to leave it to the surgeon and not get involved directly, at least until the surgery is over!

However, expecting a doctor to fix you is generally a bad idea. The role of a physician is to diagnose the condition of your health and act as a catalyst for your healing by suggesting remedies and directions, and treating you with appropriate therapies.

Healing is an inside job and you are the star of the show. Only you have the power to heal your body. No physician, remedy, or treatment has the power to heal you unless your innate capacity to heal cooperates. All of the healing arts are about helping your body heal itself.

Your involvement in the process is vital because what you do for yourself on a daily basis to support (or jeopardize) your health has more to do with the state of your health in the long run than any physician, treatment, or medicine. Regardless of who you have on your team to help you support your health, you, and only you, are ultimately in control of your own health.

No one can do as good a job nurturing and protecting your health as you. No matter how good my doctoring is, my patients don't get well by my actions alone. No matter how good my doctoring is, I know the people I work with can't get well by what I do alone. Without their involvement, I know the results they get will be partial or short-lived. That's just the way it is.

More money is spent on health care in the United States per person than any country in the world. We are spending more money all the time to come up with new drugs, surgeries, and treatments. Yet, our health as a whole isn't that much better for it. The problem is that the standard model of medicine doesn't require self-responsibility.

Only you are with you all the time. Only you can control the conditions that create the state of your health. Don't abdicate this job to someone else — even your doctor. Only you can do the job right.

Produce Measurable Results

Functional Medicine has value because its results are measurable. It's important to be able to measure how your body functions and what results you get from any therapies you use.

Using the scientific model in functional selfcare looks like this: test your body functions, determine what the findings mean, apply the indicated therapies, and retest your body functions to determine the outcome. Using this strategy, you will always be able assess the effectiveness of any therapy by the results.

Individuals and Environments are Interdependent

People and their environment are completely and mutually interdependent. The ecological approach in healthcare sees these relationships and understands that the environment, both natural and human, must be healthy to have healthy individuals. Practitioners of the healing arts have a responsibility to promote healthy and ecologically sound environments that are sustainable and that nurture the full expression of life in all its manifestations.

Use a Global and Long-Term View

Supporting your health needs *now* will create an environment that will support your health in the future. In Functional Medicine — preventing illness by maintaining health and solving health problems before they create symptoms — is preferred. Often, when treating symptoms by using traditional forms of medicine, the long-term effects on your health or the effects on your health as a whole aren't considered

Functional Medicine considers your health as a whole and for the future. This includes considering how a therapy affects other body systems apart from the system directly associated with symptoms, and how a therapy may reflect on your long-term health.

The Principles of Healing

I am repeating some of the ideas from the previous section on Functional Medicine, but I feel that presenting the basic principles of how your body heals, separately from the ideas about Functional Medicine, will be useful.

When I refer to healing, I am speaking about the process of your body healing itself from within and becoming well.

The Principles of Healing

- Your body is naturally self-healing.
- Resolve cause to restore function.
- Balance the triad of health as a whole.
- Healing is a process.

Your Body is Naturally Self-Healing

Natural forces are the healers of disease. ~ Hippocrates

There is a vital force, an innate intelligence, inherent to all living things. Your innate intelligence works to heal and regulate your body. In other words, it is your natural state to be self-healing, self-regulating, well and vital, and to fully express your inherent strengths and gifts. Science calls the expression of this principle *homeostasis*.

Resolve Cause to Restore Function

Find it, fix it, and leave it alone. ~ Clarence Gonstead, DC

To get well and stay well you have to treat the cause of a symptom or dysfunction. Treating symptoms can be useful in the short run, but will never get you well. Treating symptoms, for instance, by getting an epinephrine shot if you have a severe asthma attack can even save your life. However, by treating the symptom and not the cause, you can pretty much count on having to treat for the same symptoms into the future. It's like fanning smoke and never putting out the fire.

Resolving cause, however, is an extremely efficient way of restoring your health. Once the cause for a health problem is eliminated, the myriad symptoms associated with the underlying health problem will tend to resolve spontaneously.

Balance the Triad of Health as a Whole

Anything can cause anything. ~ Lance West, DC

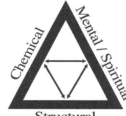

Your body is an incredibly complex and completely integrated system. The Triad of Health is a model that acknowledges the interplay and interconnectedness of your structural, chemical, and mental/spiritual aspects.

All aspects of the triad of health must be considered, and all relationships between the aspects of the triad of health included. These various aspects are part of a unified whole. The parts of the whole are actually one.

If you have a headache, you can take aspirin or some other pain-reliever. But a pain-reliever is just that — a *pain*-reliever. It's useful in the short run, but what about headaches that keep coming back? You don't need a pain-reliever then. You need a *cause*-reliever.

If you have any kind of ongoing or reoccurring pain, taking pain-relievers is like painting over rust; the rust (problem) is still there underneath the coat of paint, and it will just keep popping up through the paint (the pain-reliever).

You have to get to the cause to solve a health problem. Until you do, you'll be managing your symptoms but never solving the problem. Headaches, for instance, can be caused by neck (spinal) subluxations, jaw (TMJ) or tooth problems, cranial bone problems (indicating the need for craniosacral therapy), foot problems, pelvic problems, and shoulder dysfunction.

And that's just a partial list of things that can cause headaches from the structural side of the Triad of Health.

On the chemical side, headaches could be caused by liver dysfunction, allergies, Vitamin B deficiency, digestive dysfunction, imbalances of the flora (normal bacteria) in your gut, mineral imbalances, dehydration, hormonal imbalances, and deficient saturation of oxygen in your tissues. That's a partial list. Then, of course, emotional stress with its cascade of effects could be the cause, too. Using the Triad of Health helps us to understand that the cause isn't necessarily in the same place as your symptoms.

Healing is a Process

We've been trained to believe that the answer for most health problems is a specific pill, potion, or procedure and that we should be "fixed" pretty much right then and there, or at least within a few days. Your body can heal itself on that kind of schedule, but not always.

Very severe or very chronic health problems take time for your body to heal. Healing is a process, not an event. Drugs and other medicines can change symptoms rapidly, but healing may not coincide with the change in symptoms.

When looking at the effects of many medicines (drugs), it can look like your body can be fixed instantaneously. What is often taking place, though, is that your body is being forced to function in certain ways by the action of the drug. The effect is only present as long as you take the medication. The underlying process causing your symptoms is still present.

That's not to say that drugs are never appropriate. They are useful for managing symptoms and they often can resolve cause. A good example is antibiotics. When prescribed at the right time and for the right reasons, antibiotics can solve the cause of an infection. Recurrent infections, however, are not caused by bacteria, but rather by weakness of your immune system.

If weakness of your immune system were the underlying reason for recurrent infections, antibiotics would only provide a temporary solution. You'd still be open to most every bug you were exposed to. The only way to get over getting everything that comes around would be to strengthen your resistance to infection.

Another good example of treating symptoms is using antiinflammatory medications to treat pain. To use medication like that once in a while is no big deal, but if you need to use it all of the time, it's not a real solution. You need to look elsewhere to solve the problem.

Look for the underlying causes to find real solutions. Address the cause, restore function, and give yourself time to heal. Be patient and know in the long run you'll be way ahead of the game.

This workbook will have absolutely **zero** impact on your health if you only read it. For these profoundly powerful tools and methods to make difference, you have to go beyond the reading and get to the doing part. These pages are full of information to make you stronger, healthier, and more vital. All of this might seem a little intimidating at first. Don't worry. As you go through the process, it will all come together.

The last thing I want for you is for this workbook to be a "shelf-help book," one you bought to improve your life but ends up sitting on the shelf unused. The workbook you have in your hand is powerful; the tools within it can change lives. I know this with certainty, because the strategies found here come from my practice and I see miracles in people's lives from using them. Reading this workbook and making use of the many tools it offers will be life-changing and life-affirming for you.

Have you ever worked on a paint-by-the-numbers painting? When you first look at the picture, it looks like a mess of squiggly lines that don't look like they could possibly end up being a picture. But, you start painting each field according to the color indicated by each number. You don't see the picture yet, but you trust the process. You don't have to know what you're doing. All you need to do is paint each number the right color. Then suddenly, magically, you see it! You see the picture. You didn't have to know what you were doing; you painted a picture anyway.

Using this workbook is just like that. You don't have to know what you're doing, and it doesn't have to make sense when you start out.

Leap in, start doing it, and go through the process. Just like painting-by-the-numbers, all of a sudden you'll see the picture: you'll get it.

Using this workbook is much like learning to ride a bike. Initially you struggle a bit, but then there comes a moment when you begin to get a feel for it, and from that point on, everything else gets easier. As you work with the information presented, trust that you will develop that same feeling and understanding for the process.

The good news is that it's hard to go wrong when you're using lifestyle and nutritional approaches.

Use the guidelines in this workbook. Use common sense. Follow the guidelines for when you need a physician. Be sure to keep him or her informed, especially if you're taking prescription medications.

You can read the whole workbook cover-to-cover and then begin the health graph, home exams, and lab interpretations. You also have the option of going immediately to filling out the forms and following the suggestions for improving your health.

You can use this workbook on an as-needed basis. When some health problem comes up, you can pull it off the shelf to find a solution.

The real power of this workbook, however, comes from using it regularly.
Being really healthy is much like being really fit, in that exercise and nutrition must be part of your daily routine. It is not fulfilled by the occasional healthy meal or the every-now-and-then workout.

Functional Selfcare Overview

THE FUNDAMENTALS: THE ELEMENTS OF HEALTH

- Breathing
- Water
- Salt
- Foundation Diet
- Non-Toxic Environment
- Detoxification and Fasting
- Exercise
- Sleep, Rest, and Relaxation

- Being Present and Doing Nothing
- Recreation (Play)
- Moderation
- Meditation, Contemplation, and Prayer
- Relationships
- Mission and Purpose
- Contribution

THE SPECIFICS: SELF-DIRECTED FUNCTIONAL SELFCARE

Health Graph	Blood Tests	Home Tests

- Compile results and support yourself accordingly.
- Reevaluate periodically.

- Health Graph and Home Tests every 2-12 weeks.
- Lab Tests every 6 weeks to 12 months.

Keep using these tools regularly to know your health status and direct your functional selfcare.

The Elements of Health represent the fundamental components of your lifestyle that support your health and well-being.

You can use any combination of the Health Graphs, Home Tests, and Blood Tests. They each stand alone, even though they are synergistic when used together.

Strategies for Choosing Health

LEARNING STYLE
Use the style that's right for you.

SEEING

1. Look to the flowcharts in Using the Workbook.
2. Flip through the tables and flowcharts to get an overall view of the major concepts and strategies.
3. Earmark pages you know you'll want to read or reference later.

DOING

1. Get a feel for the Workbook by completing a Health Graph.
2. Experiment with any of the Elements of Health.
3. As you use and understand the strategies, develop a program that best supports your active learning style.

READING

1. Read the entire book to get a good understanding of the tools and concepts.
2. As you read, use a highlighter to mark any information you feel will be instrumental in your self-care.
3. Re-read everything you've highlighted for an overview.

The Elements of Health

● **Breathing**	Full oxygenation of your body is essential to vitality.
● **Water**	Hydration allows optimum function of each cell of your body, balanced body chemistry, and detoxification.
● **Salt**	Electrolytes (salts) provide the polarity in charge required for metabolism, nerve conduction, and cell membrane transport.
● **Foundation Diet**	Needed for your body to repair and regenerate itself; provides the energy from which to take action.
● **Non-Toxic Environment**	Eliminates stress on your body from toxic chemicals.
● **Detoxification and Fasting**	Eliminates accumulated wastes from metabolism and toxins (mostly chemicals) from your body.
● **Exercise**	Maintains strength, flexibility, and coordination; increases blood and lymph flow; oxygenates your body.
● **Sleep, Rest, and Relaxation**	Needed by your body and mind to repair and regenerate; provides the energy from which to take action.
● **Being Present and Doing Nothing**	Reconnects the body, mind, and spirit as one and affirms we are more than what we do.
● **Recreation (Play)**	Provides pleasure and reconnects body, mind, and spirit; source of inspiration and insight.
● **Moderation**	Gives freedom and happiness through being without addictions and dogma; encourages compassion.
● **Meditation, Contemplation, and Prayer**	Connects life with values; gives meaning, understanding, and direction; creates relaxation.
● **Relationships**	Provide a sense of connection and a place in life; a source of support, love, inspiration, example, and guidance.
● **Mission and Purpose**	Gives a sense of importance (reason for being), direction, and reference points for accomplishment.
● **Contribution**	1) Contribute to others and yourself through giving whenever an opportunity to do so arises. 2) Have one or more areas to which you focus on making a contribution, i.e., donating time and/or money to charities, mentoring someone, being a Big Brother or Big Sister, etc.

The Elements of Health in Relation to The Triad of Health

ASPECT SUPPORTED

Chemistry	Structure	Mind and Spirit
• Breathing	• Sleep, Rest, and Relaxation	• Being Present and Doing Nothing
• Water	• Exercise	• Meditation, Contemplation, and Prayer
• Salt		• Moderation
• Foundation Diet		• Recreation (Play)
• Non-Toxic Environment		• Relationships
• Detoxification and Fasting		• Mission and Purpose
		• Contribution

The Elements of Health listed above are arranged not only according to which side of the Triad of Health they support, but also according to their hierarchy of need.

The most immediate needs are listed at the top. This gives you a focus to work first on the elements that are highest on the list. As you are able to incorporate an element into your life, work on the next element.

For Mind and Spirit, it may seem curious I put the element of Relationships so far down on the list but the elements that go before it create ways of being which increase your ability to relate more fully and harmoniously.

Incorporating The Elements of Health: Chemistry*

- **Breathing**
  1) Practice as outlined in The Elements of Health: Breathing for 2-10 minutes, 1-2 times a day.
  2) Periodically take note of your breathing, noticing its quality; practice breathing techniques briefly to reinforce the technique.
  3) As you incorporate natural and complete breathing into your daily life, decrease your practice to a few times a week.

- **Water**
  1) Drink approximately as many ounces of water a day as are equal to half your body weight.
     (Example: Your weight is 160 lbs, you should drink 80 oz of water a day)
  2) When you drink enough water throughout the day, your urine will be clear; adjust your intake upward if your urine is not clear.

- **Salt**
  1) Use Celtic salt liberally in your diet, while avoiding commercial salt and foods containing commercial salt.
  2) Adding ½ tsp of salt, 1-2 times a day may help replenish electrolytes depleted by past use of commercial salt, exercise, or chronic stress.

- **Foundation Diet**

  With anything you eat or drink, ask:
  1) Is this food or drink in its natural and unrefined state?
  2) Is this food or drink cooked or raw?

- **Non-Toxic Environment**
  1) Evaluate your environment for the presence of toxins and eliminate as many of them from your environment as possible.
  2) Look to soaps, shampoos, toothpastes, lotions, and cosmetics as a possible source of toxins.
     (See Environmental Resources in The Elements of Health: Non-Toxic Environment.)

- **Detoxification and Fasting**
  1) Use fresh vegetable juices daily.
  2) Consider fasting on water or juices once a week.
  3) Use a fast or cleanse 2-6 times a year.
     (See Detoxification and Fasting: Putting It All Together for direction.)

* Listed by hierarchy of need.

Incorporating The Elements of Health: Structural

- **Sleep**
  1) Assume you need 8 hours of sleep a night.
  2) Get some exercise a few hours before bed (walking is sufficient).
  3) Decrease the light you are exposed to at night.
  4) Use reading, meditation, contemplation, and/or prayer before bed.
  5) Go to bed at approximately the same time every night.
  6) Retire earlier in the night to improve the quality of your sleep.

- **Rest and Relaxation**
  1) Have relaxing and pleasurable routines in your life.
  2) Take time to enjoy yourself alone and in the company of others every day.

- **Aerobic Exercise**
  1) Train 3-6 times a week for 20-40 minutes.
  2) Track your heart rate. (See Aerobic Training in The Elements of Health: Exercise.)

- **Anaerobic Exercise**
  1) Weight train 3 times a week (intense calisthenics are an acceptable alternative).
  2) Do compound movements (use more than one joint at a time).
  3) Ideally, use free weights (barbells, dumbbells, and cable machines) and/or bodyweight training (chin-ups, dips, etc.).

- **Flexibility Training**
  1) Prior to exercise, do warmup and light stretching to prevent injury; afterward, stretch to increase flexibility.
  2) Stretch daily from 10-20 minutes (more is great).

- **Neuromuscular Training**
  1) Look to how you can incorporate (stimulate) your nervous system more fully during any training.
  2) Use some coordination-focused activity daily (i.e., juggling, dancing, etc.).
  3) Experiment with new and different activities to exercise your nervous system, discover unexplored capacities, and maintain coordination as you age.

- **Energetic Training**
  1) Use Tai Chi, Chi Gung, yoga, Tibetan yoga, or martial arts daily.
  2) Train once or twice a day for 10 minutes or more.

Incorporating The Elements of Health: Mind and Spirit

- **Being Present and Doing Nothing**
  1) Make note of when you are acting unconsciously or are disassociated from the present moment, and bring your consciousness to the present moment.
  2) Give yourself time daily for doing nothing (activity having no particular purpose).

- **Meditation, Contemplation, and Prayer**
  1) Meditate for 10-20 minutes, 1-2 times a day.
  2) Spend time in contemplation and prayer daily.

- **Moderation**
  1) Ask: *Is there reason present in what I think and do?*
  2) Exercise compassion moment-by-moment with yourself and others.
  3) Whenever you experience suffering (discomfort or unhappiness), determine the addiction causing it; determine the thwarted pure intention and act to fulfill it directly.

- **Recreation (Play)**
  1) Recognize the possibility of spontaneously creative being (play) which is present in essentially any moment.
  2) Give yourself time daily to practice.

- **Relationships**
  1) Realize that in every moment alone or with others, relationships are present.
  2) Be conscious of the qualities of relationships through the questions from The Elements of Health: Relationships.

- **Mission and Purpose**
  1) Determine your mission and purpose using the questions from The Elements Of Health: Mission and Purpose.
  2) Determine and acquire the skills needed to manifest your mission and purpose through introspection and study (formal and informal).

- **Contribution**
  1) Contribute to others and yourself through giving whenever an opportunity to do so arises.
  2) Choose a mission (or missions) upon which you focus.

The Specifics: Self-Directed Functional Selfcare

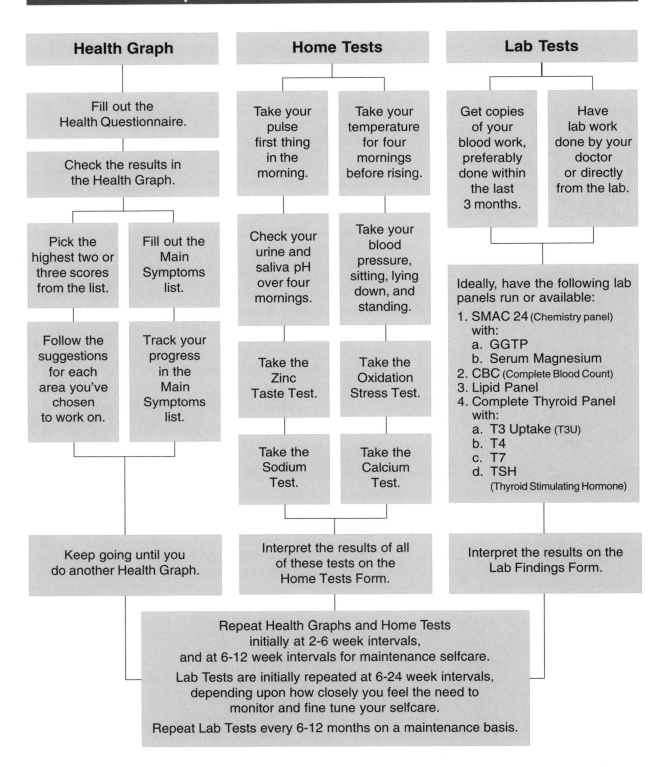

Health Graph

Fill out the Health Questionnaire.

Check the results in the Health Graph.

Pick the highest two or three scores from the list.

Fill out the Main Symptoms list.

Follow the suggestions for each area you've chosen to work on.

Track your progress in the Main Symptoms list.

Keep going until you do another Health Graph.

Home Tests

Take your pulse first thing in the morning.

Take your temperature for four mornings before rising.

Check your urine and saliva pH over four mornings.

Take your blood pressure, sitting, lying down, and standing.

Take the Zinc Taste Test.

Take the Oxidation Stress Test.

Take the Sodium Test.

Take the Calcium Test.

Interpret the results of all of these tests on the Home Tests Form.

Lab Tests

Get copies of your blood work, preferably done within the last 3 months.

Have lab work done by your doctor or directly from the lab.

Ideally, have the following lab panels run or available:
1. SMAC 24 (Chemistry panel) with:
   a. GGTP
   b. Serum Magnesium
2. CBC (Complete Blood Count)
3. Lipid Panel
4. Complete Thyroid Panel with:
   a. T3 Uptake (T3U)
   b. T4
   c. T7
   d. TSH (Thyroid Stimulating Hormone)

Interpret the results on the Lab Findings Form.

Repeat Health Graphs and Home Tests initially at 2-6 week intervals, and at 6-12 week intervals for maintenance selfcare.

Lab Tests are initially repeated at 6-24 week intervals, depending upon how closely you feel the need to monitor and fine tune your selfcare.

Repeat Lab Tests every 6-12 months on a maintenance basis.

Glossary

Code	Meaning
Primary Support	● Most important nutritional support
Secondary Support	● Second most important nutritional support
Tertiary Support	● Third most important nutritional support
*** Source	● Best source
** Source	● Second-best source
* Source	● Third-best source
BID	● Twice a day
TID	● Three times a day
QID	● Four times a day
d	● drop
D	● Full dropper
mmHg	● Millimeters of mercury; a standard of measure for blood pressure.
tsp	● teaspoon
Tbsp	● Tablespoon
B	● Bottle
Generic	● Nutritional support is generally available at health food stores; manufacturer or source isn't critical.
AHC	● Made by Amazon Herb Company
BRC	● Made by Biotics Research Corporation
DR	● Made by Dragon River
KAL	● Made by KAL
SPL	● Made by Standard Process Labs
YP	● Made by Yerba Prima
Generic/BRC	● Different sources are equivalent and will be equally effective.

Dietary Supplement Sources

Company	Abbrev	Available From	Phone Orders
● Biotics Research Corp.	BRC	DSD International	800-232-3183 602-944-0104
● Amazon Herb Company	AHC	Amazon Herb Company	800-835-0850
● The Synergy Company	TSC	The Synergy Company	435-259-5366
● KAL	KAL	Health food stores or	
● Yerba Prima	YP	*The Elements of Health*	
● Dragon River	DR	*The Elements of Health*	866-563-4256
● Standard Process Labs	SPL		theelementsofhealth.com

Note: Any of these products may be available directly from doctors endorsing and incorporating the *choosing* HEALTH system with their patients.

General Principles

Regardless of the state of your health, certain fundamental elements must be present in your life for you to have good health. These fundamentals comprise the Elements of Health.

The Elements of Health are much like the elements from the periodic table; the elements of health can be bound together in a multitude of ways, creating an infinite variety of outcomes.

As you experiment with the elements of health covered in this workbook, you will experience the results and can use this information to fine-tune how you use them. You will find you have control over your health. You can even use different combinations and emphasize certain aspects of the elements of health to support your life in ways that work for you. In that way, the elements of health can be used to help you create a life that suits you.

These things comprise the essential elements of selfcare that must be present for you to be healthy, **in my opinion**.

What I am presenting here comes from almost twenty years of working with people to help them solve their health problems and be healthier. In every case, the people I've worked with who have had poor health have had a deficiency or imbalance of one or more of these elements, and that very issue was causing or contributing to their illness.

By contrast, those people who have had a very high level of health tend to have a good balance of the elements of health in their lives.

Using the elements of health to support your health gives you greater ability to adapt to the stresses (physical, chemical, and emotional) that are present in your life. When you are able to adapt to your environment, you are well, and when you are unable to adapt to your environment, you are ill.

By using what you know about the elements of health to control your environment and strengthen your ability to adapt, you can be in control of your health.

Those things that comprise the elements of health are listed on the next page. Each element will be expanded upon in the rest of this section. They are not written in stone; they are, rather, my opinion and feelings based on working 25 years with the question, "What are those ingredients that make for a healthy, rich, and full life?"

These are intended as a guide for exploration. I invite you to discover elements not listed here that will add to your health and wellbeing. Toward that end, you are likely to find the bibliography at the end of this workbook useful.

Breathing

Breath is life. There is no other element of health more important than the breath. As important as breath is to life, to health, and to vitality, most people don't know how to breathe effectively.

Most people have been taught that they should suck in their belly and breath high into the upper part of their chest. This is profoundly limits breathing. By breathing this way, your vital capacity — the amount of air your lungs can work with, is dramatically limited — and your energy and endurance suffers. Breathing this way causes imbalances in the autonomic nervous system, resulting in nervousness, anxiety, and depression while simultaneously hindering digestion and elimination.

Natural breathing optimizes energy and endurance, creates poise and calm, massages the organs of the abdomen to improve circulation and tone, and thereby improves digestion and elimination. Natural breathing also improves and maintains flexibility of the spine, pelvis, and rib cage through the rhythmic movement of these structures that occurs with full, natural, and unrestricted breathing. Natural breathing directly improves athletic performance.

Circulation throughout your body is improved with natural breathing, through increased circulation in the lymphatic system and increased oxygenation of the blood and tissues. Your body becomes less affected by cold when you breathe fully, and your hands and feet will feel warmer. Because of improved oxygenation and circulation to your brain, your thinking will be clearer and faster and your spirits will improve.

So what is natural breathing? It is the breathing of a child before he or she has been taught differently. It is full and unrestricted and involves movement of your abdomen (belly), pelvis, spine, and ribcage. With this inclusive movement of your body with each breath, your lungs are free to expand fully and function optimally.

Inhalation

- Inhale through your nostrils (nose).
- Let your abdomen (belly) expand.
- Let your ribs expand and your chest rise slightly.
- Let your pelvis rock forward and downward.
- Let the floor of your pelvis relax and expand slightly.

Exhalation

- Exhale through your nostrils.
- Actively contract your abdomen, including the muscles in the sides of your abdomen.
- Contract your ribcage; even contract the muscles between your ribs.
- Your pelvis rocks backward and upward.
- Contract the floor of your pelvis.

Initially, practice standing with your feet shoulder-width apart and your knees slightly bent. Place your hands with your index and middle fingers meeting on the lower part of your abdomen just below your umbilicus (belly-button). Follow the directions as above, focusing on the rocking movement of your pelvis and the expansion of your abdomen. When done properly, you will feel a slight stretching sensation in your sacrum (back of your pelvis).

This represents natural breathing, which will dramatically improve your health. Setting aside 10 minutes once or twice a day to focus on the process will soon make this way of breathing feel quite natural to you.

Here are some tips:

- When breathing in, imagine the air is coming in through your umbilicus (belly-button).

- Take note of your shoulders — if you're using your diaphragm fully and breathing efficiently, your shoulders will stay level.

- If you're having trouble getting a feel for breathing into your abdomen, practice lying on your back. Put a book or some other object on your belly and practice pushing it up toward the ceiling when you breathe in.

- You may feel a little dizzy because your brain isn't used to the increased oxygen.

- You may experience a vague nausea when first starting this practice. It represents a shift and increase in your level of energy.

- If you have trouble breathing through your nose, consider you may have trouble with allergies. Look to the Allergies section of the Health Graph and follow the recommendations. The most common reason for problems breathing through your nose is nasal congestion from milk and/or grain allergies. If you're having trouble with nasal congestion, avoid milk and milk products (except butter) and grains (pasta, bread, pastries, etc.) for a week or two to see if your congestion clears up.

Water

Water is life. Fluids other than pure water don't act the same as water in your body, and they don't meet your needs for hydration like water does. Most people are slightly dehydrated from relying on other fluids besides water for their fluid intake. Coffee, tea, and sodas even dehydrate your body.

Dehydration commonly causes fatigue, constipation, headaches, indigestion, muscle and joint aches and pains, asthma, allergies, high blood pressure, depression, diabetes, strokes, high cholesterol, tinnitus, vertigo, hearing loss, glaucoma, cataracts, and many other symptoms and diseases. To understand more fully the profound effects of dehydration, Dr. Batmanghelidj's book, *Your Bodies' Many Cries For Water,* is brilliant. His website, *www.watercure.com*, has many articles and resources.

Water quality, progressing from the ideal to the acceptable, is distilled/carbon-block combination, distilled, reverse-osmosis filter, spring/well when from an uncontaminated source, pressed carbon-block filter, granular activated-charcoal filter. Use distilled water whenever possible; it is far and away the best water for you.

Drink a lot of water! In fact, whenever you are thirsty or hungry, reach for water first to see if that satisfies you. Carbonated water with essences of natural flavoring (i.e., lemon, lime, orange, etc.) is fine and functions in your body like plain water. Juices, teas, etc., are fine, but should only be considered as an addition to your water requirements.

Drink as many ounces of water every day as are equal to half your body weight in pounds (e.g., body weight 150 lbs. = 75 ounces water a day). Use more water in hot weather and with heavy exercise. When you're actually drinking enough water, your urine will be essentially clear.

When taking B vitamins, you can expect your urine to be alternately clear and not clear. It is normal for Vitamin B2 (riboflavin) to turn your urine a very bright yellow, and at other times of the day, it will be clear.

You can check your hydration on your lab work. (See Using Lab Tests: Hydration.) Another way to make sure you're hydrated is the Skin Turgor Test. Pinch the skin on the back of your hand between your thumb and index finger, pull it away from your hand, and let go. Your skin should instantly snap back. If there is any lag, you're dehydrated. If you're testing dehydrated despite drinking a lot of water, you either need to use (more) Celtic salt, or balance your adrenal gland function. (See Stress and Life and The Health Graph: High Adrenal and Low Adrenal.)

Many digestive problems, joint and muscle aches and pains, problems with fatigue — even your complexion — will clear up with the use of more water, especially when you get rid of the sodas, milk, coffee, etc. as sources of fluids at the same time.

It's okay to drink some water with meals, because digestive enzymes are hydrolytic. That's a fancy way of saying they're activated by water. So drinking a little water with meals is good (4-8 ounces, depending on the size of the meal). The bulk of the water you drink throughout the day, however, is best taken between meals.

Salt

Salt has had considerable impact on past civilizations. Salt has been used as currency, and wars have been fought over control of salt supplies. The salt tax in France may have brought on the French Revolution.

Roman soldiers were given a salt ration because Roman generals knew their men needed salt for strength, endurance, intelligence, and courage. Today, animal breeders know the vital importance of salt and always make sure it is available to their animals. Athletes know how important salt is to their performance and ability to recuperate after exercise. Yet salt has been labeled as a health hazard; the cause of high blood pressure, heart attacks, and strokes. Many doctors today recommend not using salt at all.

The salt you use today is not at all the same salt of yesterday. Standard table salt causes imbalances between the different types of electrolytes (sodium, potassium, magnesium, and chloride).

The charge in electrolytes provides the spark that powers the cells of your body, allowing the transport of nutrients into your cells and the elimination of waste products from them. Without electrolytes there is no circulation, muscle contraction, or even nerve function. The right salts used in the right ways are the greatest inhibitors of aging; cell repair and rejuvenation depend upon adequate salt (saline solution). Standard table salt upsets the balance and causes abnormal function throughout your body. This is true even for most salt bought at the health food store.

One of the problems with commercial table salt is that by the time you get it, all of the wonderful minerals that were present originally have been extracted to be used in the chemical industry. For instance, the salt industry removes the magnesium prior to selling it for consumption, because the magnesium is used in making explosives. The selling of minerals to chemical plants is more profitable to the salt industry than the sale of the salt to you. Yet historically, salt-making was considered an art, the most distinguished artisans being the Celts.

The Celtic peoples were a very innovative race who dominated nearly all of Western Europe at one time. They perfected the methods of salt-making through the use of evaporation ponds and based much of their trade on selling and controlling salt. The last remaining Celtic salt flats are in Brittany, France. The approximately 9,000 acres of salt ponds are a national preserve. Here water is channeled in to shallow, clay-lined ponds where sun and wind evaporate the water, and the salt crystals that settle to the bottom of the pond are harvested with wooden rakes. Other than some sun-drying at this point, no other processing is done. This rich Celtic salt has 84 different elements not present in regular salt, such as iodine, zinc, magnesium, manganese, and chromium.

Possible Signs of Natural Salt Deficiency

- Brittle bones and osteoporosis
- Abnormal mineral deposits in tissues (arteriosclerosis, cataracts, kidney stones)
- Malabsorption of nutrients from food
- Abnormal muscle function such as cramping, spasm, and chronic tension (includes heart function)
- Poor glandular function (adrenal glands, thyroid, male/female organs)
- Poor nerve functions
- Kidney problems
- Edema
- Incontinence
- Chronic back pain
- Poor circulation
- Heaviness or fluid in the lungs
- High or low blood pressure
- Sugar cravings
- Joint stiffness
- Heartburn and/or sour stomach
- Masculinization of females and feminization of males
- Tendency towards addictions
- Depression
- Low sperm count or female infertility
- Chronic urinary tract infections
- Constant urination and/or profuse sweating
- Constipation
- Lack of appetite
- Gas, bloating, and indigestion
- Eating raw foods causes stomach pain
- Menstrual irregularities
- Decreased sexual desire
- Low stomach hydrochloric acid
- Marked fatigue
- Anorexia
- Nausea
- Abdominal cramps
- Insomnia

Using Celtic Salt

Dietary

Use Celtic salt on foods as you would regular salt. You may find it to be stronger than regular salt and may not need to use as much. You may find that once you taste it and start using it, you will crave it quite heavily for awhile before naturally tapering down. This is probably your body realizing it needs the salt.

Cook the salt as little as possible. Add to food at the end of cooking or, best, at the table. This salt brings the flavor out of foods, whereas the use of regular salt deadens the sense of taste.

Men seem to need more salt than women. During puberty, pregnancy, and menopause, women have increased need for iodine and may benefit from using more salt at these times.

Vegetarians need more salt to help with the digestion of vegetables. Often, vegetarians can eliminate trouble with gas and bloating by using Celtic salt.

The iodine in natural salt seems to be better utilized and tolerated than the iodine found in other sources. Celtic salt fortifies a body under increased stress by aiding the function of the adrenal glands. Many people find they are calmer, stronger, and have more courage. Many people notice being more clear-headed when using this salt. This salt can even help a person recover more quickly from shock.

Supplemental

You can supplement your diet with the light gray Celtic salt to build up the minerals in your body more quickly than is possible by using salt only in your diet. This wouldn't be necessary if we had always eaten whole foods and natural salt. The use of refined foods depletes the minerals your body needs to function optimally.

Take ¼ to ½ teaspoon of Celtic salt in water or dilute juice once or twice a day. Because the salt is cleansing, you may experience flu-like symptoms and/or nausea, fatigue, rashes, and other symptoms. This cleansing process is very beneficial to your health in the long run, but if it becomes too uncomfortable, decrease the amount of salt you are using. Taking too much salt may make you feel over-stimulated, nervous, or compulsive.

Bathing and Washing with Celtic Salt

The minerals in Celtic salt are also absorbed through your skin. Most people feel a marked improvement in their energy, decreased tension, and improved skin tone and complexion when using salt baths.

Bath salt bought in large quantities is cheaper than the standard light gray. Use approximately four cups in a large tub of warm water. This high concentration of salt forces the minerals across your skin and into your system. If the water is too hot, it will actually leach minerals from your body. Warm water allows better absorption of the minerals in the salt.

Brushing your skin with a vegetable bristle brush before the bath dilates your pores to aid mineral absorption. After the bath, don't rinse; rather, lightly towel yourself dry. The best time to use the salt bath is when you get up; a salt bath before going to bed can be too invigorating and prevent you from sleeping.

Washing your face with Celtic salt dissolved in water can be wonderful for clearing your complexion. It is very useful for chronic acne and a blotchy complexion. Wash your face with the saltwater solution and let it dry on the skin.

Brushing your teeth with a mixture of Celtic salt and baking soda will improve the health of your gums, keep your teeth free of tartar, and brighten your teeth.

Types of Celtic Salt

- **Light Gray** — The standard salt; for use on foods and as a supplement.

- **Flower of the Ocean** — Delicate, feminine; balances female hormonal levels.

- **Marine Matrix** — Seawater solution that replenishes extracellular fluid and restores mineral balance.

- **Bath** — Unwashed light gray salt; cheaper than the standard light gray when used for bathing.

The Grain and Salt Society, www.celtic-seasalt.com, 800-867-7258, carries a very coarse Celtic salt; I highly recommend you break it down using a salt grinder designed for Celtic salt, available from the Grain and Salt Society as well. The grinder has a ceramic surface that works beautifully and does not clog.

Foundation Diet: Getting Past Food Fads

General Principles

Today's food is tomorrow's you. ~ *Harry Eidenier*

Many of my patients are frustrated with the amount of conflicting diet information they've been getting. Yet there are some basic, simple, and reliable guidelines.

Use these recommendations as tools. Don't be dogmatic about them. It is best to be persistent and gentle with yourself when working toward a better diet. You don't have to be perfect, and you don't have to change overnight. Usually a slow movement toward a better diet is the one that lasts.

The following recommendations are general and will support your health overall. They don't cover the particulars of diets that may be indicated for you from the specific and self-directed processes which appear later in this workbook.

Principles of the Foundation Diet

- Eat natural foods in their natural and unrefined state whenever possible.
- Eat between 50–75% of the foods in your diet in their raw, uncooked state.

Following these two simple principles will vastly improve the quality of your diet. These principles are extremely practical to implement. Before you eat, ask yourself:

- Is this food in its natural and unrefined state?
- Is this food cooked or raw?

Eat natural foods in their natural and unrefined state whenever possible.

Dr. Weston Price, while on sabbatical from his practice of dentistry, traveled around the world researching the health status of native peoples when raised on their traditional diet, and when raised on a diet of refined and processed foods. His observations are recorded in the classic and brilliant book, *Diet and Physical Degeneration,* available from the Price-Pottenger Nutrition Foundation or The Weston A. Price Foundation. (See <u>Appendices: How to Find Functional Medicine Doctors</u>.)

Dr. Price found, measured, and substantiated a marked degeneration in the health status of native peoples throughout the world when living on a diet of refined food. This degeneration is most likely attributable to the absence of many nutrients in processed foods, especially trace minerals. Dr. Price found little variation in the health of various native peoples around the world when they ate their native diet, regardless of the diet's composition. According to Dr. Price's findings, as long people eat unrefined foods, they'll enjoy robust good health. This is eloquently and succinctly stated by Jack LaLanne when he says, "If man made it, don't eat it!"

Dr. Price's findings were recently substantiated by a report in the medical journal *The Lancet* by physicians observing the effects of modern diet in relation to a native diet among Australian aborigines.

Another issue with regard to using natural foods is the addition of chemicals to our food. Chemicals are to be avoided whenever possible, as they are without doubt health-destroying.

Harmful Chemicals in Foods

- Antibiotic and steroid residues in beef, pork, chicken eggs, milk, and milk products.
- Insecticide residues in fruits, vegetables, and grains.
- Flavorings, colorings, preservatives, etc.
- Hydrogenated or partially hydrogenated oils, especially margarine.
- Artificial sweeteners (especially Nutrasweet).
- Genetically modified organisms (GMOs) — foods that have been genetically altered.

Note: Though technically not a chemical, the effects of GMOs are stressful to the body, and research indicates there may well be long-term effects on your health.

Consider buying organically grown foods. Organic foods are free of pesticides and other harmful chemicals are higher in essential vitamins and minerals than commercially grown produce. In addition, no chemicals are used in the growing to be left in the groundwater and to affect animals and plants in the environment.

Organic animal products (beef, chicken, pork, fish, milk, cheese, butter, eggs, etc.) are particularly important. Because the residues from pesticides and other chemicals (including toxic metals) become more concentrated as they travel up the food chain, concentrations of these toxins are higher in animal products than in produce and grains.

If you must choose between purchasing organic produce and organic animal products, buy the organic butter, milk, meats, etc. Butter is an excellent food when it is part of a whole-food diet, and it is particularly important to get this food organically produced.

Eat 50–75% of the foods in your diet in their raw, uncooked state

This recommendation comes from research done by Francis Pottenger, MD, who evaluated the health of different populations of cats raised on raw versus cooked diets.

What Dr. Pottenger observed in the cat population living on a cooked-food diet was the development of degenerative diseases (such as allergies, arthritis, asthma, thyroid disorders, increased incidence of birth defects, stillbirths and spontaneous abortions, osteoporosis, osteoarthritis, heart problems, near- and farsightedness, bronchitis, decreased resistance to infection, parasites, lack of normal sexual maturation, gum disease, tooth loss, and decreased life span) that worsened every succeeding generation until the population was unable to reproduce. Dr. Pottenger then took some of these degenerated cats and established a regenerating population fed on raw food, and this population then became fully healthy, with genetic expression to match the initial raw-food population.

Dr. Pottenger concluded that cooking foods breaks down the proteins and enzymes present in raw foods. He felt these factors were critical for the repair and maintenance of the body. Raw foods tend to be rich in enzymes.

Here is a list of raw protein-rich foods:
- Raw or rare meat (beef is the safest; don't eat rare ground meat).
- Raw eggs (the risk for Salmonella is extremely low if you use cage-free, fertile eggs).
- Raw nuts and seeds, and raw nut butters.
- Sprouts of all kinds (this includes sprouted-grain breads).
- Raw milk and milk products (like raw cheese).

In my daily diet, I eat raw nuts and seeds rich in essential fatty acids. I also eat good-quality, rare meat and raw eggs a few times a week. The eggs can be blended in juice (orange juice is the best), or in milk with a touch of honey (makes a wonderful eggnog).

I feel stronger and have more energy when I have these raw proteins in my diet. Both the Price-Pottenger Foundation and the Weston A. Price Foundation (Appendices: How To Find Functional Medicine Doctors) have a lot of information and recipes on including more raw protein in your diet.

Recommended Foods

Most people's diets contain too few vegetables and too many grains in the form of breads, pastas, and sweets. Eating fewer grains and more vegetables will significantly improve your diet.

Testing your saliva and urine pH is the most accurate and dynamic way to modify the Foundation Diet to your specific needs. This is covered in Using Home Tests: Body pH. Foods shown below in bold are particularly recommended.

Grains
Brown rice, steel-cut **oats** (not quick or rolled oats), millet, buckwheat, barley (hulled, not pearled), rye, cornmeal, wheat.

Beans and Legumes
Pinto, black, **garbanzo**, azuki, black-eyed peas, lima, **soy**, lentils, kidney, split peas, peanuts, cashews.

Nuts
Almonds, pecans, filberts, **walnuts**, chestnuts, Brazil, pinon, coconut, cashews.

Seeds
Sesame, sunflower, **pumpkin**, **flax**, chia, psyllium.

Vegetables
All vegetables are recommended. Be creative and use some of the exotic vegetables like Chinese cabbage, dulse, kelp, nori, and jicama.

Fruits
Apples (especially green), pears, peaches, grapes, guava, **papaya**, mango, oranges, **lime**, **lemon**, grapefruit, **pineapple**, apricot, plum, melons, dates, **figs**, tangerines, all berries, bananas, tangelos, and actually any I have not mentioned.

Herbs and Spices
Celtic salt, fresh-ground pepper, **garlic**, **onions**, **cayenne**, **ginger**, parsley, basil, sage, turmeric, curry, bay, cardamom, coriander, cumin, dill, fennel, marjoram, mustard, oregano, paprika, cinnamon, nutmeg, rosemary, saffron, tarragon.

Dairy Products
Whole raw milk, raw cheese, yogurt, kefir, **butter**, **fertile eggs**.

Meats
Organic (if at all possible) beef, pork, chicken, fish, shellfish, lamb, turkey.

Oils
Flax, **extra virgin olive**, **sesame**, almond, avocado, corn, **wheat germ**, safflower.

Sweeteners
Honey, maple syrup, barley malt, raw cane sugar (Succanat®) and stevia.

Vinegar
Balsamic, **apple cider**.

Sample Menu

Upon rising: Large glass of water (with fresh squeezed lemon, lime, or orange, if you prefer) and tea *or* fresh fruit or vegetable juice.

Breakfast: Fresh fruit, nuts, yogurt, or kefir, a cooked-grain cereal, if desired, *or* eggs, meat, and vegetables.

Eggs are an excellent food with an unjustifiable bad name. They are an excellent protein source, especially when you buy eggs from hens raised cage-free (or range-fed) and chemical-free. Fertile eggs have a higher nutrient value than regular eggs.

Experiment with breakfast. Some people do best with fruit, raw nuts, juice, and water until lunch. Using this program can make a tremendous difference in your energy, digestion, and elimination. This type of breakfast is used by many of the traditionally long-lived peoples; it may be a factor in longevity. Others do best eating more concentrated foods like grains and proteins for breakfast.

The heavier breakfast program is usually best for those who have a mid-morning drop in energy, usually due to fluctuating blood sugar. Use each program for a week, take note, then use the one that feels best for you. Morning hunger is normal. If you don't have a morning hunger, eat a smaller and earlier dinner. Your stomach and other digestive organs will thank you.

Lunch: Large salad, casserole, or meat, soup, bread once in a while (with butter, if desired), nuts, cooked vegetables (including potatoes), cottage cheese, or cheese.

Dinner: Similar to lunch.

Snacks: Fruit, raw vegetables, nuts, small slice of cheese, etc.

Foods to Avoid in Your Diet

- **Hydrogenated oils (including margarine)**
- **Sugar and white flour and anything made with them**
- Excessive use of coffee or black tea, sodas and soft drinks
- Candies and chocolates
- Excessive alcohol
- Commercial salt
- Foods that have been refined, flavored, and colored
- Rancid or spoiled foods (especially oils)
- Meats, eggs, and dairy products from animals raised with antibiotics and steroids

If you are consistently working with your diet and generally staying within the guidelines as listed above, you will enjoy wonderfully improved health even though you occasionally eat foods from the above list. Your desire for these foods will lessen as you improve your diet. Just for reference, I have wine, beer, coffee, ice cream, and even candies and pastries once in a while.

What you do most of the time is what matters the most. I'm convinced many people make themselves sick by being overly obsessive about their diet. Eating a healthy diet isn't about being obsessive or suffering or doing without a life. A healthy diet is about enjoying life (including food and drink) and feeling healthy, vital, and strong. A healthy diet affirms and celebrates life.

About Dietary Supplements

Dietary supplements are important because the foods we eat usually don't contain many critical nutrients. This is due to depleted soils, food refining, and polluted environments. Our needs for many nutrients are increased because of environmental pollution and excessively stressful lifestyles.

Don't nickel-and-dime yourself to death with a cupboard full of vitamins. I commonly see people who are taking so many supplements their body doesn't know what to do with itself. Supplements are just that—supplements to your diet. Primarily, use a good multiple-vitamin and -mineral supplement that emphasizes the trace minerals. The most common nutrient deficiency I see in practice is of trace minerals. For a listing of vitamins, minerals, and trace minerals, see Appendices: Using Food To Balance Body Functions.

Below are dietary supplements I consider the basics. It's rare for people to not notice a significant improvement in their health when taking these formulas. Most people using these multiple vitamin/mineral formulas and antioxidants consider them the best they have ever used. These are "industrial-strength" and are usually only available through physicians.

Basic Dietary Supplements

Primary Support: Multiple-vitamin/mineral formula

Iron, and Copper-Free Bio-Multi Plus (BRC)

Take 3 tablets a day. It is best to divide the dosage by taking one tablet per meal, or two in the morning and one at night. Take with meals or at least some food, because the zinc sometimes upsets an empty stomach. Use regular Bio-Multi Plus instead if you are a cycling female or test for iron-deficiency anemia from your red blood cell count (RBC).

Secondary Support: Antioxidant Formula

Bioprotect (BRC)

Antioxidants decrease the biochemical stress on your whole body, improve function overall, improve resistance, decrease inflammation and pain, and decrease degenerative diseases associated with aging if taken over a long period of time. This is a very balanced formula and is much more effective (and less expensive) than taking the antioxidant nutrients separately. Take one to three capsules a day.

By taking formulas rather than individual vitamins and minerals, you save yourself money and the trouble of mixing and matching individual bottles. Minerals and vitamins work ideally in certain ratios to one another, and this has been worked out for you. These formulas are very reasonable in cost, especially considering the quality. These are the formulas I recommend for my patients. Bio-Multi Plus, Iron, and Copper-Free Bio-Multi Plus, and Bio-Protect are available from DSD International, 800-232-3183 or 602-944-0104.

Basic Dietary Supplements: Food Concentrate and Herb-Based Support

Supplement	Ingredients
Pure Synergy Powder	**Algae Blend:** Spirulina; blue green algae, chlorella, dunaliella, kelp, bladderwrack, and dulse (contains more protein, iron, Vitamin B12, trace minerals, RNA, DNA, chlorophyll and beta-carotene by weight than any other known natural food source); **Chinese Mushrooms and Herbal Blend**: reishi, shiitake, maitake, cordyceps. astragalus, ginger, schizandra, licorice root (these herbs are tonic and balance the immune and hormonal systems); **Sprout Blend** (includes plant enzymes): sprouts of millet, kamut, quinoa, broccoli, spelt; green papaya (includes the plant enzymes—amylase, cellulase, lipase, and protease); **Concentrated Green Juice Powders**: Juice concentrates of kamut grass, barley grass, oat grass, alfalfa grass (source of lutein, octacosanol, and carotenes, vitamins, trace minerals, hormone-balancing factors, plant enzymes, and protein); **Western Herbal Blend**: Red clover flower, nettle leaf, parsley leaf, burdock root, yellow dock root, skullcap flower and leaf, dandelion leaf, ginkgo leaf, and rose hips (these herbs are detoxifying and tonic); **Plant-Based Antioxidant:** extracts of rosemary leaf, clove, and sage.
Vita Synergy Tablets:	**Vitamins, Minerals and Trace Minerals plus** **Women's Formula:** Extracts of Chastetree, Shatavari, Siberian Ginseng, Brahmi, Ashwaganda, Wild Yam, Motherwort, Raspberry, Damiana, Lotus, Licorice, Hawthorn, Gotu Kola, Triphala, Amla, Bibhitake, Haritake, Turmeric, Jatamansi, Green Oat Grass, Shilaji, Ginger, Rose Petal, Lavender, Passion Flower, St. John's Wort, Magnolia, Chamomile, Calendula, Chrysanthemum, Honeysuckle, Dendrobium, Rosemary, Sage, Clove, Fennel, Cardamom, Vanilla and naturally occurring plant extracts (RNA/DNA, SOD, Glutathione, all Essential Trace Minerals, Amino Acids, Beta-Glucans, GABA, Alpha Lipoic Acid, Chlorophyll, Polysaccharides, Enzymes, Isoflavones). **Men's Formula:** Extracts of Ashwagandha, American Ginseng, Siberian Ginseng, Fo-Ti, Damiana, Wild Oat Seed, Shatavari, Brahmi, Gotu Kola, Tribulus terrestris, Triphala Fruits (Amla, Bibhitake, Haritake), Turmeric, Hawthorn, Licorice Root, Solomon's Seal, Jatamansi, Green Oat Grass, Shilajit, Ginger, Saffron, Dendrobium, Chrysanthemum, Rosemary, Sage, Clove, Fennel, Sandalwood, Cardamom, Cinnamon, Vanilla and naturally occurring nutrients from plant extracts (RNA/DNA, SOD, Glutathione, all Essential Trace Minerals, Amino Acids, Beta-Glucans, GABA, Alpha Lipoic Acid, Chlorophyll, Polysaccharides, Enzymes, Isoflavones).

Both Pure Synergy Powder and Vita Synergy are expensive, but if you have health problems and need the extra boost of these very complex food and herb concentrate formulas, or if you want extra support due to particularly stressful lifestyle, use these formulas. Each can be taken alone, though they are synergistic when taken together. Take as directed on the label. These formulas are available from The Synergy Company, 435-259-5366, www.synergy-co.com.

Non-Toxic Environment

Today you are constantly exposed to chemicals that never existed 100 years ago. This barrage of chemicals is extremely stressful to your body. It's no wonder that cancers, asthma, allergies, learning disabilities (especially Attention Deficit Disorder), depression, infertility, male and female hormone problems, cardiovascular diseases, birth defects, diabetes, Alzheimer's disease, and so many other diseases are rampant, increasing in frequency, and resistant to medicine's machinations.

Environmental Toxins

Family	What To Do
Pesticides and Herbicides	Minimize or eliminate the use of herbicides and pesticides around your home. Use pest control companies that offer low-toxicity or organic sprays. Use organic solutions for weed control.
Household Chemicals	Keep chemicals outside of the house (i.e., in the garage). Use organic alternatives.
Cosmetics, Soaps, Shampoos, etc.	Use organic alternatives.
Plastics	Buy foods in glass rather than plastic whenever possible. Keep foods in glass rather than plastic. Avoid cooking in non-stick cookware.
Molds	Minimize standing water and constant moisture and humidity that encourage mold growth in your home. Clean mold with borax. Use HEPA-rated air purifiers to keep your environment free of mold spores.
Dust and Dander	Use bedding and pillow covers that are dust-mite-proof. Use water filter or HEPA-filtered vacuum cleaners. Use HEPA-rated air purifiers.
Air Pollution	Live rurally, if possible. Exercise away from polluted areas. Use HEPA filters at home and at work. Drive less and use less consumptive cars. Use low-tech solutions to gas-powered tools like lawn mowers, leaf blowers, etc.
Industrial Chemicals	Buy fewer manufactured and more high-quality goods whenever possible; they will last longer and thereby save energy and raw materials. Support legislation requiring cleaner manufacturing practices.
Toxic Metals	Avoid metal-based dental amalgams. Avoid deodorants containing forms of aluminum. Avoid cigarette smoke. Avoid cooking in aluminum and non-stick cookware.

Minimize your exposure to household chemicals, as they tend to be very toxic. Look for natural alternatives. It's amazing how effective and inexpensive vinegar, borax, and baking soda can be for cleaning around the house.

Most cosmetics (including hair dyes and treatments) contain some of the most toxic chemicals imaginable; however, natural and non-toxic cosmetics alternatives are widely available.

Many environmental chemicals (particularly plastics and pesticides) are hormone disruptors (xenobiotics). These have a profound influence on male and female hormones and primarily mimic the effects of estrogen. It's interesting (and scary) to note that average sperm count values have gone down consistently since the 1940s. Most symptoms with regard to female hormones that women complain of have to do with too much estrogen or xenobiotics in their bodies, or too high a ratio of estrogen to progesterone.

Environmental Resources

Doris Rapp, MD	Her website and books are invaluable resources. Her book, *Is This Your Chemical World?*, is a must-read, 800-787-8780, www.drrapp.com.
Aveda	Source of non-toxic cosmetics and hair and body care, 866-823-1425, www.aveda.com.
Burt's Bees	Source of non-toxic cosmetics and hair and body care, 800-849-7112, www1.burtsbees.com.
C.A.R.E.S. for Life Foundation	The orientation of this organization is around the toxic effects of personal-care goods (shampoos, soaps, sunscreens, etc.) and cosmetics, 719-742-3310, www.toxicfree.org.
Eco Clean	Resources for household cleaning and laundry goods, air purifiers, vacuums, low-toxicity stains and paints, dust-mite-proof bedding, home test kits, and much more. They have a great catalog and are a reliable resource for information, 480-947-5286, www.ecoclean-az.com.
Gaiam, Inc.	Low-toxicity, natural sources for household goods and cleaning agents, 800-869-3446, www.gaiam.com.
Global Campaign to Reduce the Use of Toxic Chemicals	Information provided through the World Wildlife Fund. Lots of information on toxic chemicals; many website links. Fax: 202-530-0743, www.worldwildlife.org/toxics.
Morganics	This company has a great collection of non-toxic household cleaning goods, skin-care goods, nutrition, and essential oils, 800-820-9235, www.morganics.com.
EcoMall	A web-based clearing house for non-toxic resources, www.ecomall.com.

Environmental Resources *(continued)*

Natural Home Magazine	This is a wonderful resource. Very professional, rational, thoughtful, and complete, 800-272-2193, www.naturalhomemag.com.
Angelic Botanicals	I use these essential oil misters in my office instead of the standard (and toxic) air fresheners, 252-412-2008, www.angelicbotanicals.com.

Detoxification and Fasting

Detoxification

Every day we are exposed to toxic chemicals that didn't exist when our grandparents were born. We are exposed to cleansers, solvents, cleaning agents (like the formaldehyde residues in dry-cleaned clothes), pesticides, herbicides, fungicides, and other toxic agents in the air we breathe, the food we eat, and the water we drink.

Your lungs, large intestine, kidneys, skin, kidneys, gall bladder, and liver are all designed to eliminate toxins, but often your body becomes overwhelmed and your health is compromised as a result. It's no wonder you might not feel so well.

Symptoms Indicating a Need for Detoxification

- fatigue
- skin rashes
- toxic headaches
- gas and bloating
- broken capillaries
- hypoglycemia
- varicose veins
- high blood pressure
- light-colored stools

- generalized joint and/or muscle pain
- male or female hormonal problems
- muddy complexion with spots (especially along the jawline)
- venous congestion (seen as bulging veins on face and neck)
- indigestion from high-fat fried foods
- swollen abdomen or ankles
- tendency to constipation

- pasty skin
- arthritis
- allergies
- boils
- hemorrhoids
- acne
- jaundice

One of the best things that you can do to compensate for toxic environment and support for your health is to cleanse and detoxify. Easy, effective, and safe methods are available to accomplish this task. I recommend some type of cleansing regimen every three to six months long-term, and these programs can be used on a more frequent basis if you are actively working on a health problem.

When on a cleansing program, it is normal to experience fatigue, headaches, muscle and joint aches/pains, nausea, inability to concentrate, and possibly skin breakouts (acne or rashes). As your body eliminates accumulated toxins in your system, you may feel "off." Experiencing this reaction confirms that the cleanse was needed, and the result will be better health. If the reactions are too strong, decrease the dosage of herbs or use the cleanse only a few days a week. You have time; you don't have to get it all done yesterday.

Detoxification Strategies

Program	Benefit	Notes
Basic Program	A very gentle and effective general cleanse; a healthier feeling overall; regularity.	The most convenient cleansing program, as you only have to take pills morning and night; can be used long long-term.
Beet Cleanse	A very powerful cleanse that purges the bile ducts and liver; very good at increasing energy.	Methyl donors from beets can have a profound effect on energy; a powerful therapy for chronic fatigue syndrome and fibromyalgia syndrome.
Liver/Gall Bladder Purge	This is the cleanse to use if you test positive for problems with Liver/Gall Bladder in The Health Graph and Using Home Tests sections.	Chronic mild to moderate gall bladder problems can be resolved with this cleanse. If gall bladder problems are severe, consult a physician.
Juices	Provides gentle and powerful detoxification; increases energy, mental clarity, and wellbeing, decreases pain, and increases flexibility.	Compensates for lack of adequate vegetables in the diet; probably the best long-term strategy. Definitely use juicing to feel and look young!
One-Day Fast	Increases energy overall and decreases fluctuations in energy; normalizes hormone balances.	Increases growth hormone levels, normalizes blood sugar levels, improves absorption of foods in diet; a powerful long-term strategy when used weekly.
Short Fast (2-3 days)	A deeper cleansing for specific health problems or as a periodic health maintenance strategy.	Often the catalyst for healing; use when detoxification strategies without fasting don't produce results.
Long Fast (4-10 days)	The deepest cleansing for complex or severe health problems or as a periodic health maintenance measure for people very committed to optimum health.	Often produces healing when nothing else does; can profoundly improve mental clarity and insight.

Basic Cleanse

Basic Cleanse (2-6 Weeks)	
Supplement	**How To Take**
Herbal Guard (YP)	1-4 capsules or tablets BID
Colon Care (YP)	2-6 capsules BID morning and evening
Women's Renew (YP) or Men's Rebuild (YP)	1-4 capsules BID morning and evening
Optional Ingredients	
Cholacol II (SPL) *or* Hydrated Bentonite* (YP)	4 tablets 15 minutes before meals *or* 1-2 Tbsp in dilute juice BID

*Hydrated Bentonite is more effective than Cholacol II, but less convenient.

Start with a low dosage of each for a few days, and increase to the higher dosage over 4-7 days. Some people don't tolerate the higher doses and find them uncomfortable. Use the highest recommended dosage you're able to tolerate.

Herbal Guard, Women's Renew/Men's Rebuild, and Colon Care are available in a boxed set: the Women's Renew Internal Cleansing System or Men's Rebuild Internal Cleansing System. These make an excellent and very convenient cleanse. For the first time around, I recommend taking three boxes back-to-back. That will make for about six weeks of cleanse. You'll have Colon Care left over. Keep taking it until it is gone.

Benefits of the Basic Cleanse

This is a very convenient cleanse to use when the deeper-acting, but more involved cleanses are too difficult to fit into a hectic schedule. It is relatively gentle and can serve as a good beginning. This program can also be used over a long period with excellent results. This program has the same benefits as the beet cleanse, though to a slightly lesser degree.

Notes on the Basic Cleanse

If you're using the Hydrated Bentonite, start with 1 tsp BID and work up to 2 Tbsp BID over 4-10 days. Starting with the full dosage can cause constipation. Take Bentonite (including Cholacol II) separately from other supplements.

Make sure you drink a lot of water when using this cleanse.

You will most likely have more frequent stools; they will be larger than usual and more darkly colored. This is normal.

It is normal to have at least one very bulky stool a day while using this program. You may notice mucous, debris, or dark material in your stool. This is normal and shows that the program is being effective in cleansing your intestines.

Beet Cleanse

Beet Cleanse (2 to 6 Weeks)	
Ingredients	**How To Take**
Beet Mix One cup shredded raw beets Two tablespoons flax oil Juice of one-half lemon	1) Take 1 tsp every 1-2 hours for 3 days 2) Take 2 Tbsp TID for 7 days 3) Continue at 2 Tbsp BID for 4-32 days 4) The longer cleanse is the idea
Colon Plus Powder (BRC) or Psyllium Hulls (Generic)	2-8 capsules BID morning and evening or 1 tsp–1 Tbsp BID in eight ounces of water or diluted juice
Optional Ingredients Cholacol II (SPL) or Hydrated Bentonite* (YP)	4 tablets 15 minutes before meals or 1-2 Tbsp in diluted juice BID

Use Spectrum flax oil if possible. Flax oil goes rancid very rapidly, so get the smallest bottles you can and keep them in the refrigerator.

If you're using the Hydrated Bentonite, start with 1 tsp BID and work up to 2 Tbsp BID over 4-10 days. Starting with the full dosage can cause constipation. The Hydrated Bentonite can be mixed in with the Colon Plus Powder. Take these separately from other supplements.

Benefits of the Beet Cleanse

- A powerful cleanse for your liver and gall bladder
- Stimulates better digestion and elimination
- Tends to lower blood fats (cholesterol and triglycerides)
- Increases energy, concentration, and memory
- Usually resolves constipation
- Balances blood sugar
- Helps to decrease body fat
- Often profoundly powerful in restoring libido (sex drive)
- Often helpful to resolve menstrual problems (including PMS)
- Helpful for a sensitive or queasy stomach
- Resolves gas and bloating
- Clears stuffy or foggy heads
- Diminishes or eliminates muscle and joint pain or achiness
- Eliminates body odor

Notes on the Beet Cleanse

Drink a lot of water while using Colon Plus Powder. After the cleanse is finished, don't stop the Colon Plus Powder or Psyllium Hulls immediately. It is quite all right to use these bulking agents for a prolonged period, even indefinitely.

Because of the beets, it is normal for your stools to be red when you're on this program. You can also expect to have at least one very bulky stool each day while using Colon Plus Powder or Psyllium Hulls. You may notice mucous, debris, or dark material in your stool. This is also normal and shows that the program is being effective in cleansing your intestines.

Any problems encountered with Colon Plus Powder or Psyllium Hulls generally result from using too much too soon, using too much powder with too little water, not following Colon Plus Powder with an additional glass of water, or starting a program when you have serious bowel problems such as colitis or diverticulitis.

On Using Bentonite

Bentonite (from Hydrated Bentonite or Cholacol II) is very fine clay that scours debris that coats the villi of your small intestine. This coating of debris develops from eating foods that lack fiber (i.e., any refined food). By eliminating this coating from your small intestines, the full surface area of your intestines is restored and the improvement in your digestion and absorption is usually very dramatic.

There is an interesting symptom associated with this problem that very consistently indicates the need for bentonite. If you often find you feel hungry, but when you go to the fridge or the cupboard to get something to eat and can't decide what it is you want, you need bentonite.

Once you've used the bentonite for a few weeks, you will find you know exactly what you want to eat most of the time. You will also notice clearly and quickly the effects of what you eat, both good and bad, on your body.

Liver/Gall Bladder Purge

Liver/Gall Bladder Purge Preparation Phase (3-4 days)	
Ingredients	**How To Take**
• Hard, green apples (Pippin, Granny Smith)	• Eat an apple every 2–4 of hours
• Apple cider (ideally raw and unfiltered)	• Drink at least one quart a day
• Di-Sodium Phosphate (SPL)	• Two capsules three times a day
• Super Phosphozyme Liquid (BRC)	• 30 drops three times a day in water
• Colon Plus Powder (BRC)	• 2-8 capsules BID morning and evening
or	or
• Psyllium Hulls (Generic)	• 1 tsp–1 Tbsp BID in eight ounces of water or diluted juice

Liver/Gall Bladder Purge

• ½ cup of extra virgin olive oil • ½ cup of **fresh** lemon juice	Drink the olive oil and lemon juice at least three hours after eating dinner on the third or fourth night.
• One **bottle** of Coca-Cola® (room temperature)	Drinking Coca-Cola® after the olive oil and lemon juice helps control the nausea and cuts the oily taste that might be caused by the olive oil.
• Ginger root (fresh and thinly sliced)	Chewing on some fresh thinly sliced ginger root can help with the nausea and oily taste.
• Di-Sodium Phosphate (SPL)	Take two capsules before bed.

Immediately after drinking the mixture, lie down on your right side for a **minimum** of 30 minutes, with your knees drawn up to your chest.

Benefits of the Liver/Gall Bladder Purge

This cleanse is more aggressive, deeper-acting, and the results are more dramatic and immediate. You will probably experience symptoms of detoxification such as fatigue, nausea, diarrhea, acne, body odor, and headaches due to sudden mobilization of toxic debris from your system. This is a sign that the cleanse was needed.

These symptoms do not occur in people who don't have toxic systems. The good news is that these symptoms are temporary (2-4 days) and you can look forward to having greatly improved health.

Notes on the Liver/Gall Bladder Purge

Due to the effects of the apples, apple juice, and di-sodium phosphate, you may have fuller and possibly looser bowel movements during the program.

It will take about eight hours for the flush to work. You will then have a full, relatively loose bowel movement the first time.

The bulk of debris, some of which may look like small stones, will usually be eliminated with the second bowel movement. Most often you will have between 3-6 bowel movements in as many hours. Obviously, it is best to plan the flush so the day after falls on the weekend.

Taking an herbal laxative that night will help eliminate any remaining debris. An herbal laxative will also help with queasiness caused by the oil. Another solution for the queasiness that can result from the Gall Bladder/Liver Purge is to use a coffee enema as described in Detoxification and Fasting: Fasting: Long Fasts.

Juices

Fresh juices, primarily vegetable juices, help you get nutrients from fruits and vegetables in amounts sufficient to balance your body pH, restore antioxidant enzyme levels, replenish trace minerals, and detoxify the liver and lymphatic system.

Freshly made vegetable juices are best. Buy yourself a juicer. They're definitely worth the investment! Spend the extra money to get a good-quality juicer, because getting the cheapest one just means you'll end up with something that never really works right or quickly falls apart.

I recommend Acme or Omega juicers. They are very reliable and produce very tasty, pulp-free juice. If you get the Acme, get the filters for the basket, as well. The Omega juicer is a model that seems as solid as the Acme and is easier to clean. You can get both of these juicers from most health food stores or from Juicers Direct, 800-259-3023, www.juicersdirect.com.

Juice made from carrots, celery, and beets makes a great basic vegetable juice. You can add other vegetables to this as you wish, such as ginger, cucumber, parsley, spinach, wheatgrass juice, etc.

Generally, I recommend 8 to 16 ounces of fresh vegetable juice every day. This is a wonderful thing to do in support of your health. If you are working on a health problem and you want more support, use 8 to 16 ounces of vegetable juice twice a day. If you have trouble with your blood sugar because of the juice, dilute the juice with water and drink smaller amounts through the day. Or add Spirulina (generic), Blue-Green Algae (generic or TSC), or Pure Synergy powder (TSC).

The book, *How To Keep Slim, Healthy, and Young with Juice Fasting,* by Paavo Airola, ND, is a great resource for both juicing and fasting. I recommend it for further direction as you use juices in your diet and for fasting.

Wheatgrass juice is a particularly powerful food and healing agent. I recommend using wheatgrass juice, especially if you are actively working with a health problem. It will help you heal faster. Covering the growing, processing, and use of wheatgrass juice is outside the scope of this book, however. I recommend *The Wheatgrass Book* by Ann Wigmore as a guide.

Fasting

Long-lived peoples characteristically eat in moderation and fast periodically. These forms of caloric restriction have been studied extensively in lab animals and the results are very convincing: lab animals on caloric-restricted diets lived longer and exhibited fewer degenerative diseases as they aged.

I began my studies in health and healing with *The Miracle of Fasting* by Paul Bragg, ND. Dr. Bragg overcame TB as a kid with fasting, whole and natural foods and exercise. He fasted one day every week and up to a couple of weeks four times a year. He was vital and strong until the day he died in a surfing accident at 93. For him, fasting, above all else, restored his health and kept him vigorous. I recommend Dr. Bragg's book for guidance and inspiration when fasting. It has helped me immensely.

At one time, Dr. Bragg had popularized the practice of fasting one day a week among many people. I've had the pleasure of working with some of Dr. Bragg's disciples over the years and have been impressed with their overall health, vitality, looks, and strength relative to their age. I am convinced, both through my own experience and observing others, that fasting works.

A weekly fast of 24–48 hours as an ideal health maintenance measure as are periodic fasts (usually once a season) from three days to a week. This type of food restriction has been used in laboratory animals to increase the lifespan of some test groups by as much as 150%, with a coincident decrease in degenerative diseases.

The One-Day Fast
Weekly fasting makes a huge difference in my health when I have the discipline to do it. I have more energy, strength, endurance, and mental clarity. Growth hormone typically decreases with age, and there is a lot of research indicating that low growth hormone accounts for most of the things we attribute to aging. Fasting is a powerful stimulant to growth hormone levels, and that may account for a lot of the positive effects of fasting.

Ideally, fast for 24–36 hours once a week. The 24-hour fast is from dinner to the next dinner. If you want to fast for 36 hours, fast from dinner on one day, through the next day, and until breakfast on the third day.

Best results, in the long run, are when you fast on water only or on water with fresh lemon (you can add a little maple syrup). If you have difficulty fasting on water only, use fruit and/or vegetable juices, water, and herb teas as desired. Juices are preferably freshly made, but if this is not possible then glass-bottled, unpasteurized, unfiltered is a good second. Freshly made juices are much different than bottled and are much more effective.

For some, undiluted juices may cause a drop in blood sugar. If you have symptoms, especially problems with energy and/or concentration when using the juices undiluted, mix the juices with an equal amount of water.

Short Fasts (2-3 days)
Fasts of two or three days are done the same as the one-day fast, except most people use juices in addition to water.

Blue-Green Algae (generic or TSC) or Spirulina (generic) can also be used a few times a day to keep your energy levels up during the fast.

When you conclude a one-day fast, it's okay to make the first meal a regular meal. When you fast for two or more days, break the fast with a lighter-than-normal meal. The best first meal after you fast is fruit or a vegetable, such as salad with an oil and vinegar-based dressing. All meals after that, eat as you normally would.

Long Fasts (4-10 days)
Longer fasts usually work best with a few days to a week of preparation by increasing the use of raw fruits and vegetables and decreasing the use of animal products in your diet. Juices, teas, and water are the same as for the shorter fast.

With longer fasts, I recommend adding a daily enema with a pint of freshly brewed (not decaf) coffee in water. Use a knee chest position and retain as much of the coffee mixture as possible for 5-15 minutes. The reason for the coffee enema is to purge the liver and gall bladder and to loosen impacted fecal material from the colon wall so it can be eliminated.

Also effective, but not required, are the following: Colon Plus Powder (BRC; 1 tsp–1Tbsp BID) and Cholacol II (SPL; 6 tabs BID) or Liquid Bentonite (Yerba Prima; 1 tsp–2 Tbsp). This combination is to be taken 2-6 times a day with Colon Plus Powder mixed in a jar with a lid in dilute juice. You can experiment with the dosage and the frequency to find out what works best for you. When using the Liquid Bentonite, you can mix it in dilute juice with the Colon Plus Powder.

Blue-green algae (generic or TSC), Pure Synergy powder (TSC) or spirulina (generic) can be used a few times a day, also, to keep your energy levels up during the longer fasts. Take the blue-green algae, spirulina, or Pure Synergy separately from the Colon Plus Powder.

When you end a longer fast, it is best to transition to a normal diet according to the following format:

Day 1 – Fruit only
Day 2 – Add vegetables
Day 3 – Add grains, beans, nuts, seeds, and oils
Day 4 – Normal diet

Using Detoxification and Fasting

For Optimal Health
↓
Consider using 8-16 oz. of fresh vegetable juices once a day.
↓
Consider fasting one day a week on water or juices.
↓
Consider fasting
3-10 days, 2-4 times a year.
or
Use the Basic Cleanse
2-6 weeks, 2-4 times a year.
↓
If you want a deeper cleanse, use the Beet Cleanse once or twice a year.
↓
Note: Effect of the Beet Cleanse can be deepened by using the Liver/Gall Bladder Purge on the 2nd and/or 4th week.

For Resolving Health Problems
↓
Use 8-16 oz. of fresh vegetable juices once or twice a day.
↓
Fast one day a week on water or juices.
↓
Fast
3-10 days, 4 times a year.
or
Use the Beet Cleanse
with the Liver/Gall Bladder Purge on the 2nd and 4th week.
↓
As an option to the Beet Cleanse and fasting, use the Basic Cleanse continually for up to 6 months.

Fasting is not appropriate while pregnant or nursing.

Exercise

Research showns that life expectancy is determined more by exercise and fitness than any other single factor. I have often been struck by how important exercise is in relation to many of the other elements of health. So many times over the years, I have seen people who enjoy a level of health far beyond their years, simply because they exercise regularly.

Exercise Distinguished by Function

- **Aerobic** — Promotes fitness of the cardiovascular system
- **Anaerobic** — Promotes muscle size, strength and power
- **Stretching** — Promotes flexibility, circulation, speed, power and resilience
- **Neuromuscular** — Promotes integration of muscles with the nervous system
- **Energetic** — Promotes the storage and movement of life energy

Aerobic Exercise

Aerobic exercise is any exercise that forces your muscles to use more oxygen to produce energy. Aerobic exercise doesn't overwhelm your body's ability to deliver the oxygen your muscles need to function, and it builds muscle endurance and cardiovascular fitness.

Benefits of Aerobic Exercise

- Improves health of your heart and blood vessels
- Improves lymphatic circulation
- Increases oxygen levels in your body (including your brain)
- Increases the rate of metabolism (helps burn body fat)
- Increases energy, mental clarity, and sense of wellbeing
- Decreases total cholesterol while increasing HDL levels (HDL protects your heart and blood vessels)
- Lowers high blood pressure
- Releases endorphins
  (increases relaxation and wellbeing, decreases stress, and prevents depression)
- Improves blood sugar regulation
  (helps to prevent and/or control hypoglycemia, insulin resistance, and diabetes)

It doesn't matter what you do to increase your heart rate for cardiovascular aerobic fitness, the heart rate is everything.

Aerobic Training: How To Do It

- Calculate your maximum heart rate by subtracting your age from 220
  (i.e., if you're 50 years old, your maximum heart rate would be 170 (220-50 = 170)).
- Train aerobically 3-5 days a week at 60% to 90% of your maximum heart rate
  (i.e., 170 x .6 = 102 and 170 x .9 = 153).
- Track your pulse rate periodically while exercising by resting your fingers on your wrist on the same side as your thumb or in the slight depression to each side of the front of your neck. To calculate the beats per minute (bpm), count for fifteen seconds and multiply the count by four.
- If you're a beginner, stay in the lower range while exercising (60-70%).
- Once you're feeling more fit and recovering from your exercise more quickly, you can train in the higher range (80-90%) for short periods.
- Interval training is using cyclical bursts of exercise in the 80-90% range for short intervals. This kind of training powerfully increases aerobic capacity and fat-burning.
- If you are **very** fit, you can train at or above you maximum heart rate in short intervals.
- If you have major health problems or any reservations about your basic cardiovascular health, see a physician or certified physical trainer or therapist to establish your ability to train and monitor you.

For a wonderful reference on aerobic and weight training, I highly recommend a book by Clarence Bass, *Challenge Yourself At Any Age*, available by calling 505-266-5858 or www.cbass.com. His website has fantastic articles as well.

You may find that using a heart rate monitor is easier for keeping track of your heart rate than using a watch to check your pulse. Some heart rate monitors allow you to program your workouts and keep you at your target heart rate. Alarms remind you when your heart rate is outside of the target range. Polar makes the best heart rate monitors. The Polar Protrainer XT® is a heart rate monitor model designed to help you interval train. You can usually find these in sporting goods stores, or contact Polar at 888-337-4684.

Anaerobic Exercise

Anaerobic exercise is any exercise that overwhelms your body's ability to deliver adequate oxygen for your muscles to produce energy. Heavy weight training, sprinting while running, cycling, swimming, and difficult calisthenics are anaerobic exercises. Muscle failure is often the result. Anaerobic exercise increases your muscle size, strength, power, and speed, tendon and ligament strength, and promotes some cardiovascular fitness.

Benefits of Anaerobic Training

- Increases strength
- Improves posture
- Maintains and even increases bone density
- Maintains and increases muscle mass
- Decreases body fat
- Improves the aesthetics of body contours and tone
- Decreases the likelihood of injuries and helps you recover more quickly from injuries
- Improves mood and sense of wellbeing and deceases stress
- Increases metabolism

Growth hormone levels typically decline with age, closely correlated with other signs associated with aging such as muscle wasting, osteoporosis, thinning of skin, hair and nails, decreased vision, loss of vitality, and slower rates of healing from injuries or overtraining. Anaerobic exercise, especially heavy weight training, is the most powerful tool you have to keep growth hormone levels high as you age.

Testosterone increases with anaerobic exercise, particularly during exercise with a heavy barbell and dumbbells for less than 30 minutes. Testosterone is important for men and women. Women produce and need less testosterone than men, but the presence of testosterone maintains bone density, muscle mass, rate of metabolism, sex drive, mental focus, and vitality in both men and women.

I've observed over the years that people who exercise with heavy free weights for many years tend to look much younger than their age. If you're older, you have a lot to look forward to from weight training. The gains from weight training, in terms of increased percentage of strength, are usually greater for people older than 60 than for people in their 20s.

Weight Training: How To Do It

- Train your whole body three or more times a week. (Stick to three times a week at first.)

- Ideally, use barbells, dumbbells, cable weights, and exercises that use your body weight for resistance (dips, chins, and calisthenics). If you've never weight-trained, begin with machine weights for the first 4-12 weeks.

- Use movements requiring use of more than one joint at a time (compound exercises). Examples are squats, lunges, deadlifts, lat pull-downs, rows, pull-ups, dips, etc.

- Initially, use three sets of 3-12 repetitions for each movement. As you become stronger, lift more weight for three sets of three to six repetitions for each movement.

- Use weights that you can barely lift for the number of repetitions you intend to do. Stop short of muscle failure. Rest briefly between each set of exercises.

- You can put your exercise routine together so you alternate the muscles you use for each exercise (i.e., after doing a pull-up (pulling exercise), do dips (pushing exercise), then go back to the pull-ups, etc.). This is called a superset, and it allows you to get your workout done in less time and with more effect.

- Work out for no longer than 40 minutes. (It's better at less than 30 minutes.)

I highly recommend *Power to the People* by Paul Tsatsouline. This book offers a very efficient workout requiring only a single barbell. Tsatsouline also has two books on the most effective workout I have ever done: kettlebell training. They are: *The Russian Kettlebell Challenge* for men and *From Russia With Tough Love* for women. Another excellent reference for functional strength training is *Renegade Training for Football* by Coach Davies. All are available from Dragon Door Publishing, 800-899-5111, www.dragondoor.com. Another wonderful book for effective integration of aerobic and weight training is *Challenge Yourself At Any Age* by Clarence Bass. (See Aerobic Exercise table for contact info.)

If you've never weight-trained before, please use a certified trainer. Using a trainer will help you get oriented, help you get the results you're after, and keep you from getting hurt. After you feel comfortable with the weights, you have the option of working out on your own. Share the table above with the trainer, so that your exercise program can be structured around these concepts.

Flexibility Exercise

Stretching is a vitally important part of your fitness and exercise. Most people underestimate the importance of stretching.

Benefits of Flexibility Exercise

- Increases your muscle speed and power
- Improves your coordination
- Creates body and body motion symmetry
- Allows your muscles to function more efficiently from awkward positions and throughout their range of motion
- Protects your joints from injury and from the wear-and-tear type stress that results in osteoarthritis

To increase your flexibility, it is best for you to stretch *after* other forms of exercise. Warming up your body with light aerobic exercise prior to other kinds of exercise helps prevent injury, but to have any lasting effect on your flexibility, generally focus your flexibility work at the end of your workouts.

Flexibility Training: How To Do It

Types	Resources	
Standard (Easy-Hard)	Book:	*Stretching for Everyday Fitness* (SO)
	Video:	*Stretching, The Video* (SO)
Yoga (Easy-Hard)	Local:	Yoga Classes
	Book:	*How to Use Yoga* (Mira Mehta)
	Video:	*Yoga for Beginners* (LA) and *Yoga Basics* (YT)
Tai Chi Qi Gong (Easy)	Local:	Tai Chi Classes
	Books:	*Step-by-Step Tai Chi* (Lam Kan Chuen)
		The Way of Energy (Lam Kan Chuen)
	Videos:	*Vitality Qi Gong, Bliss Qi Gong, Power Qi Gong,* and *Serenity Qi Gong* (DDP)
Proprioceptive (Hard)	Book:	*Relax Into Stretch & Superjoints* (DDP)
	Video:	*Relax Into Stretch, Superjoints, & Forced Relaxation* (DDP)

SO	Stretching Online	www.stretching.com	800-333-1307
DDP	DragonDoor Publishing	www.dragondoor.com	651-644-5676
LA	Livingarts	www.livingarts.com	800-254-8464
YT	Yoga Zone	www.yogazone.com	800-264-9642

I highly recommend yoga-style stretching because of how yoga emphasizes the flexibility of your spine, as well as your shoulders, hips, etc. Yoga is a very logical approach to stretching, as all of the cardinal movements of your spine are used: flexion, extension, rotation, side bending, and long axis extension (stretching your spine lengthwise).

Tai Chi and its relative Qi Gong are very good methods for increasing flexibility if you're very stiff to begin with. Tai Chi and Qi Gong are wonderful if you're older and out of shape, or feel very weak and depleted. Both Tai Chi and Qi Gong build strength, vitality, and flexibility.

Proprioceptive flexibility training uses responses in your nervous system to help you increase flexibility. These powerful techniques are complicated at first. This kind of training has a few variations, with the most common ones going by names like Proprioceptive Neuromuscular Facilitation (PNF) and Forced Relaxation.

Neuromuscular Exercise

Neuromuscular exercise is about training for greater coordination between your muscles and your nervous system.

Benefits of Neuromuscular Exercise

- Increases the efficiency of your movement and helps your nervous system function as an integrated whole
- Improves your posture, grace, symmetry, and poise
- Increases your ability to actualize intended body action
- Increases speed and power
- Decreases your risk for injury
- Makes body movement more instinctual (subconscious)

There are a number of different activities having a neuromuscular training component to them. It's important to include exercise/training that addresses your nervous system and muscles together if you want to have a body that's at its best. Athletic performance improves and you stay more capable as you get older.

Effects by Type of Neuromuscular Training
(Grade * to ***)

Activity	Neuro-Muscular	Aerobic	Anaerobic	Flexibility
Dance	**/***	*/**/***	*/**	*/**/***
Juggling	***	0	0	*
Balance Training (tightrope/unicycle, etc.)	***	*	*	*
Gymnastics	***	**	***	***
Kettlebells	***	***	***	**
Feldenkrais	***	*	*	*
Alexander Technique	***	0	0	0
Pilates	***	**	**/***	***
Yoga	*/**/***	*/**/***	*/**/***	***
Free-Weight Training	**/***	*/**	**/***	*/**
Machine Weight Training	*	**	**	*

Mind-Body Mastery by Dan Millman does an excellent job of presenting methods for incorporating neuromuscular training into any sport, www.danmillman.com.

Kettlebells are extremely effective for neuromuscular training and build powerful, functional strength. Dragon Door Publishing, 800-899-5111, www.dragondoor.com.

Renegade Training for Football by Coach Davies is a compilation of neuromuscular training techniques and functional strength training appropriate for all athletes. Also from Dragon Door Publishing.

Energetic Exercise: Increasing Life Energy

Energetic exercise increases life energy. I define life energy as the energy reserves from which you draw as you adapt to your environment and to manifest your will in the world around you. Life energy is called Chi or Qi in China, Ki in Japan and Prana in India. The ancient Greeks called life energy Pneuma, and the French use the term élan vitale.

People with abundant life energy are able to adapt effectively to stress, handle the demands of life, stay buoyant in spirit, and display the tenacity and force of will to make their dreams and visions come true. They are strong, vital, energetic, resilient, willful, and charismatic.

Those with limited life energy aren't able to display these traits as clearly, consistently, or forcefully. There's not enough "charge in the battery" for people with limited life energy to make things happen.

Life energy, in part, is determined by genetics. The stronger the inherent genetic constitution, the more life energy the person will tend to have.

Energetic exercise is specifically focused on increasing life energy. Most energetic exercises come from the Orient, though the exercises themselves and their results are completely independent of philosophy or religion. They stand on their own merits. Examples are yoga, Tai Chi, and Qi Gong (Chi Kung).

Benefits of Energetic Exercise
(Grade * to ***)

Activity	Life Energy	Aerobic	Anaerobic	Flexibility	Neuro-muscular
Iyengar Yoga	**	*	**	***	**
Bikram Yoga	*	**	**	**	**
Ashtanga Yoga	**	***	***	***	***
Tibetan Yoga	***	**	*	*	*
Tai Chi	**	*	*	*	**
Qi Gong	***	*	*	*	**
Karate	*	***	***	**	**
Kung Fu	**	**	*	**	**

Please note these gradations are my opinion. Only a sampling of numerous energetic exercises have been included in this list. The studies of Tai Chi, Kung Fu and Qi Gong are often combined when practicing Chinese martial arts.

I highly recommend Tibetan yoga. It is fast, very effective, and needs no equipment. A book on Tibetan Yoga, *Ancient Secrets of the Fountain of Youth,* and an accompanying video are available from Harbor Press, 253-851-5190. Resources for using Tai Chi, Qi Gong, and yoga are covered in the previous section on flexibility.

Oriental martial arts, because of their integration of movement, breath, and mental focus, also function as energetic exercise. From a more objective perspective, life energy can be measured, at least in part, by measuring the symmetry and balance of resistance in acupuncture points from each meridian using an ohmmeter and with Kirlian photography. The DHEA/Cortisol Ratio from the Adrenal Stress Index Test is also a measure of life energy. (See Using Lab Tests: Specialty Tests To Consider.)

Sleep, Rest and Relaxation

Sleep

Sleep is an incredibly underestimated commodity in our fast-paced society. Sleep seems to be the first thing many of us are willing to compromise, believing that if we sleep less we can get more done. Most of the people who come to see me are sleep-deprived, and it always plays a part in the illnesses from which they suffer.

Do these things to improve the quality of your sleep:

- Assume you need at least eight hours of sleep a night.
- Get some exercise a couple of hours before bed (even a brisk walk is sufficient).
- Darkness triggers the release of melatonin and sets you up for a normal sleep pattern (circadian rhythm). Decrease the light around the house at night by using dimmer switches, lower-wattage bulbs, and even candles. Reading lights are okay if the light is focused on what you are reading.
- Minimize your exposure to microwaves, televisions, electric blankets, and plug-in radios and clocks. Electrical fields around your body decrease the release of melatonin and growth hormone that occurs shortly after falling asleep.
- Try to get to bed by 10 PM. Retiring well before midnight helps improve the normal balance of hormones that put your body into a regenerating state.
- Don't take melatonin regularly unless you've actually been tested and need it.
- Do some reading, prayer, and/or meditation — anything that relaxes you prior to bed. This will help get your body ready for sleep.

Follow these recommendations and you will start to wake up rested in the morning and notice more energy and sense of wellbeing during the day.

Life Rhythm, Rest and Relaxation

After three leaps, even a toad needs rest. ~ *Chinese proverb*

Healthy and long-lived people tend to have centering and relaxing routines and rituals to anchor them. These can be work or play or even routines of daily living. Living by routine and ritual is a very common practice in Europe.

Breaking for tea and conversation is a time-honored practice in Britain. Mediterranean peoples are known for having a long midday break for lunch (often at home), sometimes followed by a nap, before returning to the day's work. Sitting down together with family and/or friends for dinner and conversation is an effective form of relaxation. Many have prayer in church before starting the day. A walk after the evening meal is popular as well. Vacations are more frequent and longer in Europe than in the U.S., and they tend to be taken at the same time of year and to the same place.

Routines and rituals are common to cultures throughout the world and could be argued to be the definition of culture. Generally, the more sophisticated and complex the routines and rituals, the more sophisticated the culture.

Daily rituals create breaks for rest during the demands and routines of the day. Rest is created in this way throughout the day. Rest is important, because we can't always be doing; there must be time for not doing. This concept is fundamental to Chinese thought and medicine. From the perspective of Chinese philosophy and medicine, we cannot always be *doing* (yang). There must be time we are *not doing* (yin).

This concept of being both yin and yang even extends to the seasons. From Chinese philosophy, it is natural to be more active during the spring and summer when the seasons are yang. During the fall and winter, it is more natural to be more yin (less active), so our bodies can regenerate in accord with the seasons.

Examine the routines and rituals present in your life. You have complete choice as to how you create ritual and routines in your life. The point is that they nurture your spirit, provide anchoring points for the kind of life you want to enjoy, and cause you to relax. Find what works for you and enjoy more relaxation and wellbeing in your life.

Being Present and Doing Nothing

Being Present

Each small task of everyday life is part of the total harmony of the universe. ~ *St. Teresa of Lisieux*

Modern cultures encourage us to not be engaged in the present, to not be fully aware. Thinking of the mortgage, the kids, work, etc. while doing whatever we are doing as we go about our life seems natural. Yet this way of being is rare in many cultures around the world. The disconnection from life most of us tend to get caught up in, and the unhappiness and sense of emptiness that results from it, is a modern construct.

All of the distractions we commonly engage in while doing things keep us from being present; from being in the present. Yet reality is whatever moment we are currently experiencing. The past is a trace of chemical patterns in the brain, for it no longer exists. The future doesn't exist but as a mental construct, a trace of chemical patterns in the brain. Only the present exists.

Modern culture emphasizes the past and the future. The end result is that we get conditioned to believe that the past and future are more important than the present, although neither exists except as thoughts.

Living in this way, we miss our own lives because we're not there while it's happening. We may be doing things, but we miss the being that goes along with it.

This confusion is very stressful. As I have worked with people over the last twenty years, I've noticed very consistently that people who are relaxed and enjoy full and rich lives are very good at being present. They tend to live life being present to the present, and living life as it exists in the moment.

I'm not advocating giving no heed to the past and not acting in ways that provide for your future. I am advocating being present so that you're there when your life is happening.

Practice being present to what is actually occurring in each moment. Be aware of what is going on around you and inside you, in your body; how you feel and what you think. Focus your thinking around what is going on here and now.

When being present you will be aware of how rich life is each and every moment, because you will be aware of all that is actually going on and present around you. You will also notice the relaxation that naturally occurs with being present. This practice isn't limited to when you're not doing anything. Being present is something you can master at anytime, anywhere, with anyone, and while doing anything.

Doing Nothing

Give yourself time for doing nothing. Give yourself time that isn't structured or planned. Doing nothing is letting yourself be, and letting life around you be what it is.

Doing nothing is anything you do when it has no particular purpose and no required outcome.

Doing nothing can be taking a walk, luxuriating with friends and family over a casual meal, reading a book or the paper, listening to music, or lying in the grass under a tree. It is time that has no reason other than to be what it is.

Doing nothing allows you to connect with your being. Stopping and doing nothing allows us to connect more fully with the world around us and the world within us. By doing nothing, our field of vision and experience expands beyond the narrow focus of doing things for a particular purpose and reason.

Be creative; experience different places, activities, and people. Explore and enjoy yourself and the world around you. And, no, watching TV doesn't count.

Moderation

It is better to rise from life as from a banquet — neither thirsty nor drunken. ~ *Aristotle*

People who are healthy display the quality of moderation. Moderation is the expression of the attributes of reason, compassion, and emotional freedom in life. Moderation is not about being free from passion and intensity. In fact, moderation is about experiencing passion and intensity freely and fully in life. With moderation comes the freedom and ability to experience the vastly innumerable facets of life by choice.

Reason

Reason is the power of intelligent and dispassionate thought and the conduct (action) that is present due to such thought. Reason does not supercede and negate passions. Reason is much like the rider of a horse. The horse is physically more powerful than the rider, but the rider acts with will and intelligence (reason) to direct the horse's power. In this way, passions can be directed and used in ways that are desirable and constructive.

As long as your passions run in the direction you desire and choose, let them run unrestricted. If your passions run in directions you do not desire, explore them to gain insight and understanding of who you are, what you believe and value, and whether or not the aspects that make up your life are in harmony with the life you want.

Evaluating your thoughts and actions for the presence of reason is the foundation of a life that is in accord with your beliefs and values. For a more thorough exploration of reason, *Meditations* by Marcus Aurelius is the most profound discourse on the subject I have ever read. Use reason consistently in life. You will likely find as you look around (if you're like me) that there is much present in your life that is not reasonable; there is much in your life that is not in accord with your beliefs and values. Challenging yourself in this way encourages you to grow and create a more fulfilling life.

Compassion

... the goal is to develop this genuine compassion, this genuine wish for the wellbeing of another, in fact for every living being... ~ Dalai Lama

Compassion is being fully present and aware of the experience in all of its breadth and depth, in all of its suffering and sublime joy, in all of its ignorance and illumination, of being human. Compassion is being present to the human experience in others **and** in oneself. It is the awareness that all of the experiences of being human, whether inherent or manifest, are present in all of us.

We all are essentially capable of sensing, perceiving, feeling, thinking, and behaving in any and every one of the myriad of ways that comprise the human experience. Yet that doesn't translate into each of us actually doing all of the things people are capable of doing. Our feelings and thoughts may range anywhere, whereas our actions are moderated by our ethics, morals, beliefs, and reason.

We experience compassion when we are aware that we are all essentially the same, in that we are human, and that the human experience, regardless of race, culture, education, vocation, and wealth, is universal. From compassion, the qualities of love, faith, modesty, service, forgiveness, tolerance, and generosity follow naturally.

Emotional Freedom

To be addicted to anyone or anything is to be enslaved.

The presence of addiction is the absence of freedom. Where there is addiction, illusion has displaced illumination. Illumination is being aware of how you feel, what you think (and why), and what is going on around you. Illumination is being conscious of what is.

With the presence of addictions in our life we act impulsively, unconsciously, fearfully, and violently. Whenever we experience anger, fear, jealousy, anxiety, resentment, and a host of other forms of suffering, an addiction is present. Addictions are the outward manifestation of being enslaved by a belief that we must have something, someone, or some experience to occur or not occur to be happy. It is common to refer to addictions as a malevolent, external force; something that takes us over against our will.

Yet, addiction is actually not about a person, thing, or event. These all serve as objects to satisfy the addiction. Addiction is the belief that a particular internal experience (feeling) must occur or not occur to experience pleasure (happiness). Addiction is a perceived need, and solely an internal phenomenon.

The most obviously tragic problem with addictions is the compulsive, harmful actions that arise from them. Whether addictions lead to the desire for money, power, sex, people, drugs, or objects (cars, clothes, homes, etc.), they lead us to commit violence, overtly or covertly, against others and ourselves.

Where there is addiction, there is suffering (unhappiness), because addictions can never be fully or constantly satisfied. The suffering caused by our addictions leads to emotional and physical stresses that undermine our health.

Addiction is the abdication of choice, and thereby freedom. If we act from addictions being present in our lives, our thoughts and actions become structured around satisfying our addictions. The result is awareness of only those aspects of reality that threaten or support our need to satisfy our addictions. Life becomes narrowly focused and limited in scope.

Other than the physical harm to ourselves and/or others by fulfilling addictions, it doesn't matter a great deal to what we are addicted. Focusing on the addiction itself only reinforces the addiction. The solution is to focus on the process that leads to addiction.

Regardless of the suffering addictions cause, they are primarily a mental concept. The absurdity about this is that often when we experience suffering, it is only the belief we need something to stop the suffering that causes it in the first place.

Yet there is often a biochemical component to addictions, whether they range from caffeine to cocaine or chocolate to alcohol or cigarettes to antidepressants. With substance addictions, one is unconsciously or consciously trying to bring their chemistry into a balanced state. With substance addiction, I recommend using the tools in this section and help from a doctor trained in functional medicine, along with the aid of a psychotherapist and possibly support groups.

Many of the ideas here (including the basic concepts of the flowcharts below) are based on the work of Ken Keyes. His book, *Handbook to Higher Consciousness*, though a bit dated in style, is one of the most profound and seminal I have ever read.

The Structure of Suffering (Unhappiness)

Addiction **TO** have experience X	➜	Have or experience X	➜	No effect, or only short-term pleasure
	➜	Not have or experience X	➜	Suffering (Unhappiness)
Addiction **NOT TO** have experience X	➜	Have or experience X	➜	Suffering (Unhappiness)
	➜	Not have or experience X	➜	No effect, or only short-term pleasure

The pleasure experienced when addictions are present tends to be less intense and shorter-lasting, because the effect is cut short or dampened by the triggering of addictions.

Freedom from addictions means there is no absolute requirement for the experience of pleasure and happiness to occur. It doesn't mean you don't have choices or preferences for what you want in life. It does mean you don't experience suffering if your choices or preferences aren't met.

You can choose anything you want. When you operate from choice and preference, you experience pleasure every time you get what you want, and there is no effect when you don't. In this scenario, everything in your life is either a plus or neutral.

Be passionate about what you want. Have passions and powerful beliefs and commitments in your life. This is what makes for a full, rich, and well-lived life. Addictions are unrelated to all of that.

Another thing occurs when you live life with choices, rather than addictions. You realize that the filter of what would satisfy your addictions has limited your experience of life. All of a sudden, you become more aware of everything that is going on around you, and your options are greater.

This is what the model of emotional freedom looks like:

The Structure of Emotional Freedom (Happiness)				
Choose **TO** have or experience X	➜	Have or experience X	➜	Pleasure
	➜	Not have or experience X	➜	No effect
Choose **NOT TO** have or experience X	➜	Have or experience X	➜	No effect
	➜	Not have or experience X	➜	Pleasure

The pleasure experienced when exercising choices tends to be more intense and longer-lasting, because the effect is NOT cut short or dampened by the triggering of addictions.

To transform addictions into choices, ask what unexpressed or thwarted primary intention is hidden within the addiction. Thwarted and unexpressed primary intentions will always be expressed as a displaced behavior. The phenomenon of addiction is, at its core, the process of unexpressed or thwarted primary intentions resulting in displaced behavior(s). These displaced behaviors are, in their essence, perversions of one's values, however small or great, because they are an alteration and/or limitation of the primary intention.

Look to any unhappiness or discomfort (suffering) you experience and you will realize there is a belief present that you must have or not have a particular experience as a requisite for happiness (non-suffering). Reflection will help you to uncover the hidden primary intention. (See The Elements of Health: Meditation, Contemplation, and Prayer.)

Here I define intention as the emotional commitment to a desire (want). The unexpressed or thwarted primary intention that underlies the displaced behavior and addiction will always have two qualities:

- It will be true by the test of being congruent with your beliefs and values.
- The outcome of the expressed intention will cause no harm to oneself or others.

Developing Emotional Freedom

- Recognize the suffering.

- Recognize that addiction is the cause of suffering.

- Ask what the thwarted or unexpressed primary intention is that underlies the addiction.

- Ask if the intention is primary. Is it congruent to your values? And does its expression cause no harm to yourself or others?

- Determine what you need to do to be able to express the primary intention, and act accordingly.

- The cause of the addiction and the related displaced behavior resolve.

Recreation (Play)

Sell your cleverness and buy bewilderment. ~ Rumi

Recreation (re-creating) restores and regenerates the body and the spirit, and allows a break from the physical and/or mental demands of work. While relaxation is a physically passive process, recreation is an active process of regeneration.

Shifting our focus from daily demands gives the subconscious mind time to work on problems and spontaneously come up with solutions without the hindrance of our conscious mind constantly mulling them over. History is rich with people who have made discoveries, written great music, and received great insights while recreating.

Recreation is an opportunity to commune in relationships, exercise our thinking in new and different ways, learn new physical, mental, and emotional skills, uncover aspects of ourselves that we hadn't appreciated before, to have new and different experiences, to stretch ourselves, to identify our strengths and weaknesses (or yet unripened strengths), and to experience latent archetypes in our psyches, in other words, to play.

Play is also a profound exercise in being present. You can't really play and be disassociated from the present. In play, you have to be present and fully associated in body, mind, and spirit. Every part is harmonious to the whole, and there is a sense of flow, of things occurring naturally and spontaneously.

In play, as in life, spontaneity is the joyous experience of the inherent creativity of life itself. The magical experience of play is present when we abandon ourselves to it. It is in those very moments we experience a state of flow and recreation of our spirit.

Play exists sufficient in itself; it has no reason for being other than the experience of play itself. Playing is beyond our constructs about it. Play can be any action or thought you engage in solely for the enjoyment of it. I encourage you to make recreation a regular part of your life. Don't worry about what you do for play. It's all about having fun.

Meditation, Contemplation, and Prayer

Meditation

Meditation is just to be, not doing anything – no action, no thought, no emotion. You just are and it is a sheer delight…because existence is made from the stuff called joy." ~ *Osho*

With our hectic lifestyles, our need for true relaxation is great. Meditation is profoundly useful to create relaxation. Whatever preconceptions you may have about meditation, Dr. Herbert Benson's research on meditation gives great insight into how our minds control our physiology.

Dr. Benson, a cardiologist and founder of The Mind Body Medical Institute, 866-509-0732, www.mbmi.org, conducted research into the results of meditation in the 1970s. He was particularly interested in the purported cardiovascular benefits of meditation. What Dr. Benson found exceeded his expectations; in addition to cardiovascular, he found hormonal, biochemical, and emotional benefits as well. Dr. Benson's findings are distilled into his clear and insightful book, *The Relaxation Response*.

He concluded that meditation need not be a complicated or esoteric technique to work. The only requirement is a constant point of mental focus in a quiet and relaxed setting. Philosophy or religious belief is definitely not necessary to create the relaxation response.

Basic Meditation Technique

- Sit in a comfortable position in a quiet place.
- Close your eyes and pay attention to your breathing using the methods from The Elements of Health: Breathing.
- Focus your attention on the movement of your breathe: the air coming in and out, the filling and emptying of your lungs, the movement of your ribcage.
- Each time your attention drifts, come back to the focus on your breathing.
- Continue for ten to twenty minutes and do this once or (better) twice a day.
- Repetition conditions you to be in a consistently relaxed state.

Alternate-Nostril Breathing

(Usually more effective)

- Use the basic principles as from the Basic Meditation.
- Block one nostril by pushing from the side with your thumb or fingers.
- Breathe slowly and deeply pausing briefly at the end.
- Breathe out through the opposite nostril and pause briefly at the end.
- Repeat this pattern, breathing in through the right nostril and out through the left, then in through the left nostril and out through the right nostril.
- Focus on your breathing, coming back to that focus each time your mind wanders.
- Pause briefly at the end of inhalation and exhalation.

Contemplation

What lies behind us and what lies before us are tiny matters compared to what lies within us.
~ Ralph Waldo Emerson

Contemplation is reflective thought for the purpose of understanding and insight. Through contemplation you gain perspective, direction, and meaning. You come to understand the events of your life with more depth and can act in ways that are in accordance with your values and beliefs.

Give yourself time for contemplation and reflection daily. You don't need to spend a long time on it, though occasionally, when you feel particularly challenged by life, it may be helpful to do so. Usually, a few moments regarding the day will make for satisfying contemplation. This is where journaling is useful. If you haven't kept a journal before, you might want to try it. Some people find journaling very rewarding; some people would rather just spend some time in thought. Experiment and find what's valuable for you.

Prayer

Let us remember, if we want to be able to love, we must be able to pray! ~ St. Teresa of Lisieux

Daily prayer creates a relaxed state. I am making no stand for one belief over another. My experience has been that those who are truly healthy tend to believe in a higher order, and those who are ill often seem to be so because they don't have something they believe in.

By definition, prayer is directed to each individual's concept of a power greater than us which accounts for the principles and laws that create and order existence.

Prayer	
Types	**Discussion**
Petition	A prayer of petition is a request for qualities and/or characteristics for which we recognize a need to manifest more fully in our lives. These could include courage, tenacity, humility, forgiveness, wisdom, insight, understanding, tolerance, compassion, clarity, strength, calm, self-discipline, vision, and moderation. This could also be the request for a specific outcome or intercession for the success of a cause.
Confession	Recognition before God of having expressed our lives in ways that are less than our capabilities; that our actions have diverged from our ideals and beliefs. It is a realistic naming of who we have and have not been, who we are and are not, and who we can and intend to be.
Thanksgiving	Giving thanks and recognition for all we have been given; for the richness and blessings in our lives, and that all these gifts were generated from and provided by God.
Declaration	Declaring what is and what will be by the power and in accord with the will of God.
Adoration	Being in a state of love and adoration for the presence, action, and being of God.
Conversation	Having dialog with God through proclaiming our thoughts, feelings, yearnings, beliefs, dreams, and desires, and listening closely and patiently for the communication to be returned and continued.
Contemplation	Being in a state of contemplation for all that God is and for how we can be and act in accord with the being of God.
Communion	Being with the knowledge that in each moment, God is and God is present.

I make no account for what is necessarily right or true. Religious and spiritual belief is based on belief and faith and that is, and must be, a personal choice. I have discussed prayer here because of its researched effects in producing states of relaxation and my personal observations that people who are healthy tend to use prayer.

Relationships

My vocation is love...I will be love and then I will be all things. ~ St. Teresa of Lisieux

I have long noticed that good relationships coincide with good health, while the stress of poor relationships reflects in poor health. Healthy relationships provide powerful nurturing and the opportunity to nurture, allow the possibility to serve and be served, and give purpose.

Relationships call us to be ourselves, to be truthful, and to be congruent in action to belief. They let us play with being present and provide an environment to love and be loved. Relationships enrich and deepen us and make us rise up to be greater manifestations of ourselves than we would otherwise be. Use challenges to a relationship as an opportunity for growth.

The tables that follow are intended as food for thought. I hope you find them useful in making the relationships in your life more whole and gratifying.

Relationships in Life

- Self
- God (higher power/unifying principle)
- Natural World
- Mate
- Children
- Family
- Friends
- Neighbors
- Community
- Country
- World Community

Evaluating the Quality of a Relationship

- Are respect and compassion present for both parties?
- Is the relationship congruent with your values and beliefs?
- Does the relationship provide the opportunity to nurture and be nurtured?
- Is the relationship an opportunity to serve or be served?
- Is there growth present?
- Is there pleasure and even joy present?
- Is there full communication/expression of thoughts and feeling present?
- Are challenges seen as an opportunity for growth?
- Does the relationship provide an opportunity for growth?

Improving the Quality of a Relationship

- What would make the relationship more respectful, compassionate, and complete?
- What would make love and compassion present?
- How could complete communication be present?
- How could values, beliefs, vision, purpose, mission, and dreams be expressed and nurtured?

For tools to facilitate deeper and more fulfilling relationships, I recommend *Conscious Loving* and *The Conscious Heart* by Gay and Kathlyn Hendricks, 800-688-0772, www.hendricks.com. For deepening romantic relationships, *Intimate Communion* by David Deida is brilliant; 888-626-9662, www.deida.com.

Mission and Purpose

The great use of a life is to spend it for something that will outlast it. ~ *William James*

To be truly healthy and fulfilled, people need a sense of purpose, one that produces positive outcomes in other people's lives and is focused above and beyond their immediate needs and desires. Purpose gives direction to our lives and serves as a benchmark for success. Pursuing a sense of purpose forces a person to manifest capabilities and talents and provide service to others in ways they otherwise would not.

Hedonism may give pleasure, but it is almost always transient; it doesn't provide the deep satisfaction that comes from being true to an innate and unique sense of purpose. I see the lack of mission and purpose expressed as depression, melancholy, anxiety, lack of self-worth, tentativeness, addictions, anger, frustration, compulsions, and apathy.

People with a sense of purpose seem to have confidence and poise, to know who they are, and to have realistic appraisals of their strengths, weaknesses, failures, and accomplishments. They tend to be practical and effective, make things happen, and contribute to others in very tangible ways.

Determining, Clarifying, and Directing Purpose

- What things do I feel I have a talent for doing?
- What do I do that gives me the most satisfaction in life?
- Where and how do I see I could make the greatest contribution to others?
- What have I done in the past that was giving to others and that gave me a deep sense of satisfaction?

Contribution

Wherefore by their fruits ye shall know them. ~ Jesus

Healthy people sense they make a contribution to life that goes beyond their personal needs and wants. They make a difference and they know it. They know in their heart that the world is a better place because of what they have done and because of who they are.

It is easy to believe that people who have great wealth and power are the ones that make a difference in the world. In reality, it only requires the clear intention to make a difference. Essentially, everyone is presented with the opportunity to serve another person, or groups of people, every day. Every act of kindness makes a difference, makes the world better.

Here is a story that illustrates this concept beautifully:

Early one morning, a woman walks along the beach. The tide is out and there are thousands of oysters washed up on the beach from a storm the night before.

She sees a man in the distance walking toward her. He reaches down, picks up an oyster, tosses it into the surf, walks toward her again, and repeats the process.

When they meet on the beach, she asks him what difference his work will make, considering the thousands of oysters lying high on the beach in the sun.

He pauses to look at her briefly and smiles. Reaching down, he picks up another oyster and tosses it into the surf.

He looks at her again and says, "It made a difference to that one."

This is the kind of difference we can make. In each moment, through small acts, we have the opportunity to make a contribution. It doesn't matter what we do for a living or how much money we have in the bank. We all have the power to contribute to the whole and we all have the power to make a difference.

By serving others, we end up serving ourselves. The exercise of egoistic altruism serves others and makes our world more pleasurable and safer to live in.

In General

The Health Graph is a profoundly powerful tool. Besides using The Elements of Health as the foundation for your selfcare, it is the most important facet of Choosing Health. You will end up using it often, because once you learn the process, only about thirty minutes are needed to complete it. It costs you nothing and gives tremendous insight and direction to your selfcare.

I use the Health Graph on virtually every patient to guide exams and the lab work I order. The Health Graph can give me so much information that I can usually predict the lab results before I get them back. Many times, the Health Graph leads me to the real problem, even when the lab work or physical exam doesn't.

Body Systems Evaluated with the Health Graph

- Digestion
- Large Intestine
- Immune System
- Vitamin B Deficiency
- Pituitary Gland
- Adrenal Glands
- Heart

- Liver and Gall Bladder
- Allergies
- Blood Sugar Problems
- Autonomic Nervous System
- Thyroid Gland
- Nutritional Deficiencies
- Female and Male Hormones

You can get the Health Questionnaire and Health Graph Forms in the following ways:

1. Photocopy the Health Questionnaire and Health Graph Forms found at the end of this workbook.
2. Print copies of the Health Questionnaire and Health Graph Forms from the CD-ROM included with this workbook.
3. Order a packet of Health Questionnaire, Health Graph, Home Tests, and Lab Findings Forms from *The Elements of Health*, 866-563-4256.

Using the Health Questionnaire

On the next page, read each symptom and grade the following way:

Intensity of Symptom	Frequency of Symptom	Grade
Not Present	Not Present	0
Mild	Once a Month or Less	1
Moderate	Several Times a Month	2
Severe	Almost Constant	3

Your symptom merits a particular grade if it meets either the intensity or the frequency for that symptom. Look to the following table taken from a small part of the Health Questionnaire.

Health Questionnaire: Example Questions

185	Difficulty losing weight	0	1	2	3
186	Reduced initiative and/or mental sluggishness	0	1	2	3

Look at **question 185**. In this hypothetical question, intensity is the only valid criteria, so frequency isn't a concern. Grade according to whether you feel this symptom is not present, mild, moderate, or severe.

Now, look at **question 186**. Both intensity and frequency pertain. Grade according to the highest grade that fits your experience. In other words, if you feel you experience the symptom mildly but the frequency is several times a month, the grade for that symptom is based on the frequency rather than the intensity, because the frequency is of a higher grade. In this case you would grade **question 186** a **2** rather than a **1**.

Don't take too long mulling over each symptom—go with your first impression. As an example for future reference, the score for the example section from the Health Questionnaire below is **16**.

Just circle the grade for the symptoms in each section like this:

Health Questionnaire: Example Questions

185	Difficulty losing weight	0	1	2	(3)
186	Reduced initiative and/or mental sluggishness	0	1	(2)	3
187	Easily fatigued; sleepy during the day	0	1	(2)	3
188	Sensitive to cold, poor circulation, cold hands and feet	0	1	2	(3)
189	Dry or scaly skin	0	(1)	2	3
190	Ringing in ears or noises in head	(0)	1	2	3
191	Hearing impaired	(0)	1	2	3
192	Constipation	0	(1)	2	3
193	Excessive hair loss and/or coarse hair	0	1	(2)	3
194	Headache upon waking; wears off during day	0	1	(2)	3

Health Questionnaire Sample

The Health Questionnaire Forms on the following pages are for reference only.

Forms for your use are available in the back of this workbook, or may be printed from the CD-ROM included with this book.

If you have the downloaded version, all of the forms can be printed from the file.

Health Questionnaire

Name: _____ Date ___/___/___ Test #: ___

Digestion Problems

1	Bad breath	0	1	2	3
2	Loss of appetite for high-protein foods (meat, etc.)	0	1	2	3
3	Eating relieves an acid stomach	0	1	2	3
4	Gas shortly after eating	0	1	2	3
5	Indigestion ½-1 hour after eating	0	1	2	3
6	Difficulty digesting fruits/vegetables; undigested food in stool	0	1	2	3
7	Acid or spicy foods upset stomach	0	1	2	3

Liver/Gall Bladder

8	Lower bowel gas and/or bloating several hours after eating	0	1	2	3
9	Feet burn	0	1	2	3
10	Whites of eyes (sclera) yellow	0	1	2	3
11	Dry skin; itchy skin; skin peels on feet	0	1	2	3
12	Brown spots or bronzing of skin	0	1	2	3
13	Bitter metallic taste in mouth	0	1	2	3
14	Blurred vision	0	1	2	3
15	Headache over eyes	0	1	2	3
16	Feel nauseous, get queasy and/or gag easily	0	1	2	3
17	Color of stools light brown or yellow	0	1	2	3
18	Greasy or high-fat foods cause distress	0	1	2	3
19	Pain between shoulder blades	0	1	2	3
20	Dark circles under eyes	0	1	2	3
21	Acid breath	0	1	2	3
22	History of gall bladder attacks or gall bladder removed	N	—	—	Y
23	Appetite reduced	0	1	2	3

Large Intestine

24	Coated tongue or fuzzy debris on tongue	0	1	2	3
25	Pass large amounts of foul-smelling gas	0	1	2	3
26	Irritable bowel or mucous colitis	0	1	2	3
27	Alternating constipation and diarrhea	0	1	2	3
28	Bowel movements painful or difficult; constipation	0	1	2	3
29	Burning or itching anus	0	1	2	3

Allergies

30	Head congestion/sinus fullness	0	1	2	3
31	Sneezing attacks	0	1	2	3
32	Nightmares and bad dreams	0	1	2	3
33	Milk products and/or wheat products cause distress	0	1	2	3
34	Eyes and nose watery	0	1	2	3
35	Eyes swollen and puffy	0	1	2	3
36	Pulse speeds after meals and/or heart pounds after retiring	0	1	2	3

Immune System

		0	1	2	3
37	Chronic or recurrent infections	0	1	2	3
38	Constant lung congestion	0	1	2	3
39	Heal slowly from infections	0	1	2	3
40	Autoimmune disease (rheumatoid arthritis, MS, etc.)	0	1	2	3
41	Chronic fatigue syndrome and/or fibromyalgia syndrome	0	1	2	3

Blood Sugar Problems

		0	1	2	3
42	Crave sugar, sodas, or coffee in mid-morning or early afternoon	0	1	2	3
43	Hungry between meals, excessive appetite, or always hungry	0	1	2	3
44	Eating sweets upsets	0	1	2	3
45	Eat compulsively when nervous, anxious, or stressed	0	1	2	3
46	Irritable before meals	0	1	2	3
47	Shaky, weak, irritable, or light-headed between meals	0	1	2	3
48	Fatigue; eating relieves	0	1	2	3
49	Heart palpitates if meals are missed/delayed	0	1	2	3
50	Wake at night; hard to get back to sleep	0	1	2	3
51	Frequent unrealistic fears or worries	0	1	2	3
52	Often have to eat in the middle of the night	0	1	2	3
53	Often hard to concentrate or have trouble remembering things	0	1	2	3
54	Become anxious without reason	0	1	2	3
55	Excessively weak for no apparent reason	0	1	2	3
56	Often moody or depressed	0	1	2	3
57	Frequently feel drowsy	0	1	2	3
58	Difficulty making decisions	0	1	2	3
59	Often have blurred vision	0	1	2	3
60	Feel you lack sex drive	0	1	2	3
61	Often have muscle twitching or jerking	0	1	2	3
62	Feel better after eating	0	1	2	3
63	Get sleepy/drowsy after lunch	0	1	2	3

Vitamin B Deficiency

		0	1	2	3
64	Enlarged heart and/or heart failure	0	1	2	3
65	Pulse slow (below 65) or irregular pulse	0	1	2	3
66	Low blood pressure	0	1	2	3
67	Varicose veins (spider veins) and/or hemorrhoids	0	1	2	3
68	Slow reflexes	0	1	2	3
69	Irregular heart beat	0	1	2	3
70	Worry, anxiety, insecurity, or highly emotional state	0	1	2	3
71	Sensitive to noises and/or smells	0	1	2	3
72	Have trouble with concentration (foggy-headed)	0	1	2	3
73	Weak digestion (gas, bloating, indigestion)	0	1	2	3
74	Feel drowsy after eating	0	1	2	3
75	Sore and achy muscles after little exercise	0	1	2	3
76	Constantly fatigued	0	1	2	3
77	Wake up at night to urinate	0	1	2	3

78	Wake up at night and can't get back to sleep	0	1	2	3
79	Back pain when in one position (i.e., in bed at night)	0	1	2	3
80	Headband-like headache (like a tight band around head)	0	1	2	3
81	Itchy skin	0	1	2	3
82	Sensitive to insect bites	0	1	2	3
83	Shortness of breath (can't hold breath very long)	0	1	2	3
84	No stamina (get winded easily)	0	1	2	3
85	Frequently yawn	0	1	2	3
86	Low body temperature	0	1	2	3
87	Muscles feel weak (body feels heavy)	0	1	2	3

Vitamin G Deficiency

88	High blood pressure	0	1	2	3
89	Fast heart rate (pulse)	0	1	2	3
90	Muscles feel tense and tight	0	1	2	3
91	Tic-tac rhythm to heart beat (no rest between heart beats)	0	1	2	3
92	Worry excessively (mind races)	0	1	2	3
93	Always tense can't relax	0	1	2	3
94	Tend to be suspicious by nature	0	1	2	3
95	Moody	0	1	2	3
96	Depressed	0	1	2	3
97	Tend to have cold hands and feet	0	1	2	3
98	Weak digestion (gas, bloating, indigestion)	0	1	2	3
99	Muscles restless always moving	0	1	2	3
100	Body jerks when falling asleep	0	1	2	3
101	Aware of muscle twitching	0	1	2	3
102	Feel tight; not flexible	0	1	2	3
103	Trouble digesting fats (indigestion after eating fatty foods)	0	1	2	3
104	Can hear heartbeat in ears (especially lying in bed at night)	0	1	2	3
105	Cracking at the corners of mouth (cheilosis)	0	1	2	3
106	Friable, easily irritated skin (especially after shaving)	0	1	2	3
107	Red, irritated tongue (sometimes purple color to tongue)	0	1	2	3
108	Irritated mucous membranes (sinus, lungs, rectum, etc.)	0	1	2	3
109	Loss of upper lip (thin upper lip)	0	1	2	3
110	Burning or itching of eyes	0	1	2	3
111	Bloodshot eyes	0	1	2	3
112	Eyes sensitive to light (photophobia)	0	1	2	3
113	See only part of printed words (like looking through a fishbowl)	0	1	2	3

Fatty Acids Deficiency

114	Joint or muscle pain	0	1	2	3
115	Glaucoma	0	1	2	3
116	Autoimmune disease (of any kind)	0	1	2	3
117	Cold-sensitive; always feel cold	0	1	2	3

Fatty Acids Deficiency *(continued)*

		0	1	2	3
118	Chronic headaches	0	1	2	3
119	Parasthesias (abnormal sensations in body) or neuralgia	0	1	2	3
120	Muscle cramping	0	1	2	3
121	Abrupt changes in visual acuity	0	1	2	3
122	Popping or cracking in ears or tinnitis	0	1	2	3
123	Problems swallowing	0	1	2	3
124	Depression and/or anxiety	0	1	2	3
125	Learning disabilities (ADD, ADHD, etc.)	0	1	2	3
126	Epilepsy or narcolepsy	0	1	2	3
127	Dry or scaling skin (elbows, knees, forearms, shins)	0	1	2	3
128	Phyrnoderma (roughness of upper arms, thighs, buttocks)	0	1	2	3
129	Dandruff or flaking skin, in general	0	1	2	3
130	Psoriasis or eczema	0	1	2	3
131	Dyspigmentation (aging spots, vitiligo)	0	1	2	3
132	Dry or brittle hair	0	1	2	3
133	Acne	0	1	2	3

High Autonomic

		0	1	2	3
134	High blood pressure	0	1	2	3
135	Fast heart rate (pulse)	0	1	2	3
136	Dilated pupils	0	1	2	3
137	Tend toward dry mouth (may have difficulty swallowing)	0	1	2	3
138	Cold, clammy hands and feet	0	1	2	3
139	Excess muscle tension	0	1	2	3
140	Quick reflexes	0	1	2	3
141	Anxious, mind races and can't relax	0	1	2	3
142	Excessive sweating	0	1	2	3
143	Lots of energy, but poor stamina or nervous exhaustion	0	1	2	3
144	Tendency toward constipation	0	1	2	3
145	Feel like food sits in stomach; queasiness or nausea	0	1	2	3
146	Tendency toward a strong body odor	0	1	2	3
147	Women: Difficult to become sexually aroused	0	1	2	3
148	Men: Difficulty getting an erection, or weak erections	0	1	2	3

Low Autonomic

		0	1	2	3
149	Low blood pressure	0	1	2	3
150	Slow heart rate (pulse)	0	1	2	3
151	Constricted pupils	0	1	2	3
152	Tendency toward increased saliva	0	1	2	3
153	Warm, dry skin (warm hands and feet)	0	1	2	3
154	Family history of diabetes or low thyroid	0	1	2	3
155	Slow reflexes	0	1	2	3
156	Unmotivated or lackadaisical	0	1	2	3
157	Calm, even disposition	0	1	2	3

Low Autonomic (continued)

		0	1	2	3
158	Low energy but good endurance	0	1	2	3
159	Get stiff and achy after being in one position (sleeping/sitting)	0	1	2	3
160	Tendency toward laziness or undisciplined behavior	0	1	2	3
161	Women: Strong sex drive; easily aroused	0	1	2	3
162	Men: Easily achieve strong erections; strong sex drive	0	1	2	3

High Pituitary

		0	1	2	3
163	Increased sex drive	0	1	2	3
164	Splitting headaches	0	1	2	3
165	Failing memory	0	1	2	3
166	Working excessively until exhausted	0	1	2	3
167	Feeling keyed up; unable to relax	0	1	2	3
168	Reduced tolerance for sugar	0	1	2	3

Low Pituitary

		0	1	2	3
169	Reduced or absent sex drive	0	1	2	3
170	Abnormal thirst	0	1	2	3
171	Weight gain around hips or waist	0	1	2	3
172	Tendency toward ulcers or colitis	0	1	2	3
173	Ability to eat sugar without symptoms	0	1	2	3
174	Menstrual disorders (women)	0	1	2	3
175	Lack of menstruation (teenage girls)	0	1	2	3

High Thyroid

		0	1	2	3
176	Hard to gain weight despite large appetite	0	1	2	3
177	Heart palpitations	0	1	2	3
178	Nervous, emotional and/or can't work under pressure	0	1	2	3
179	Insomnia	0	1	2	3
180	Inward trembling	0	1	2	3
181	Night sweats	0	1	2	3
182	Fast pulse at rest	0	1	2	3
183	Intolerant of high temperatures	0	1	2	3
184	Easily flushed	0	1	2	3

Low Thyroid

		0	1	2	3
185	Difficulty losing weight	0	1	2	3
186	Reduced initiative and/or mental sluggishness	0	1	2	3
187	Easily fatigued; sleepy during the day	0	1	2	3
188	Sensitive to cold, poor circulation, cold hands and feet	0	1	2	3
189	Dry or scaly skin	0	1	2	3
190	Ringing in ears or noises in head	0	1	2	3
191	Hearing impaired	0	1	2	3
192	Constipation	0	1	2	3
193	Excessive hair loss and/or coarse hair	0	1	2	3
194	Headache upon waking; wears off during day	0	1	2	3

High Adrenal

		0	1	2	3
195	Increased blood pressure	0	1	2	3
196	Headaches	0	1	2	3
197	Hot flashes	0	1	2	3
198	Hair growth on face or body (females)	0	1	2	3
199	Masculine tendencies (females)	0	1	2	3

Low Adrenal

		0	1	2	3
200	Low blood pressure	0	1	2	3
201	Crave salt	0	1	2	3
202	Chronic fatigue or drowsiness	0	1	2	3
203	Afternoon yawning	0	1	2	3
204	Feeling tired upon waking	0	1	2	3
205	Weakness or dizziness	0	1	2	3
206	Weakness after colds or slow recovery	0	1	2	3
207	Poor circulation	0	1	2	3
208	Muscular and nervous exhaustion	0	1	2	3
209	Susceptible to colds, asthma, or bronchitis	0	1	2	3
210	Allergies and/or hives	0	1	2	3
211	Difficulty holding chiropractic adjustments	0	1	2	3
212	Arthritic tendencies	0	1	2	3
213	Nails weak and/or ridged	0	1	2	3
214	Perspire easily	0	1	2	3
215	Slow starter in the morning	0	1	2	3
216	Afternoon headaches	0	1	2	3

Nutritional Deficiency

		0	1	2	3
217	Frequent skin rashes and/or hives	0	1	2	3
218	Muscle cramping of leg or foot when at rest or sleeping	0	1	2	3
219	Fevers easily raised or frequent	0	1	2	3
220	Crave chocolate	0	1	2	3
221	Feet have bad odor	0	1	2	3
222	Frequent hoarseness	0	1	2	3
223	Difficulty swallowing	0	1	2	3
224	Joint stiffness upon arising	0	1	2	3
225	Frequent vomiting	0	1	2	3
226	Tendency to anemia	0	1	2	3
227	Whites of eyes (sclera) blue	0	1	2	3
228	Lump in throat	0	1	2	3
229	Dryness of eyes, mouth and/or nose	0	1	2	3
230	White spots on fingernails	0	1	2	3
231	Cuts heal slowly and/or scar easily	0	1	2	3
232	Reduced/lost sense of taste and/or smell	0	1	2	3
233	Susceptible to colds, fevers and/or infections	0	1	2	3

Nutritional Deficiency (continued)

234	Strong light irritates eyes	0	1	2	3
235	Noises in head or ringing in ears	0	1	2	3
236	Burning sensations in mouth	0	1	2	3
237	Numbness in hands and feet	0	1	2	3
238	Intolerant to MSG	0	1	2	3
239	Cannot recall dreams	0	1	2	3
240	Frequent nosebleeds	0	1	2	3
241	Bruise easily	0	1	2	3
242	Muscle cramping; worse with exercise	0	1	2	3

Heart Function

243	Aware of heavy and/or irregular breathing	0	1	2	3
244	Discomfort at high altitude	0	1	2	3
245	"Air hunger"; sigh frequently	0	1	2	3
246	Swollen ankles, worse at night	0	1	2	3
247	Shortness of breath with exertion	0	1	2	3
248	Dull pain in chest or radiating into arm, worse with exertion	0	1	2	3

Female Hormonal

249	Premenstrual tension	0	1	2	3
250	Painful menses (cramping, etc.)	0	1	2	3
251	Menstruation excessive or prolonged	0	1	2	3
252	Painful or tender breasts	0	1	2	3
253	Menstruate too frequently	0	1	2	3
254	Acne, worse at menses	0	1	2	3
255	Depressed feeling before menstruation	0	1	2	3
256	Vaginal discharge	0	1	2	3
257	Menses scanty or missed	0	1	2	3
258	Hysterectomy or ovaries removed	0	1	2	3
259	Menopausal hot flashes	0	1	2	3
260	Depression	0	1	2	3

Male Hormonal

261	Prostate trouble	0	1	2	3
262	Urination difficult or dribbling	0	1	2	3
263	Frequent night urination	0	1	2	3
264	Pain on inside of legs or heels	0	1	2	3
265	Feeling of incomplete bowel movement	0	1	2	3
266	Leg nervousness at night	0	1	2	3
267	Tire easily; avoid activity	0	1	2	3
268	Reduced sex drive	0	1	2	3
269	Depression	0	1	2	3
270	Migrating aches and pains	0	1	2	3

Using The Health Graph

Once you've completed the Health Questionnaire, graph the score for each part on the Health Graph Form. (A blank Health Graph Form can be found in the Forms section of this workbook and also included on the CD-ROM.)

Write the total score for each part of the Health Questionnaire in the appropriate box of the **Total** column; divide the resulting fraction (bottom number into top number) to come up with percentage for the **%T** column. Refer to the example below.

Make a hash mark for the resulting number in the appropriate section and use a highlighting marker to make a bar graph that looks like those in The Health Graph: Health Graph Examples.

Organ/System	Total	%T	10%	20%	30%	40%	50%	60%	70%	80%	90%	100%
Low thyroid	16 / 30	53	███	███	███	███	███					

Focus on the body systems with the top one to three scores. Most or even all of the other areas of your body that need help will get better, too. **Restoring function to the areas of your body that are under the most stress will probably fix the cause of all (or most) of your symptoms.** Go to the next section, The Health Graph: Interpreting The Results, to discover what to do to restore function to the areas of your body needing work.

To track your progress, don't forget to list your five main symptoms, in order of importance, at the bottom of the form. In the ten boxes under Percent Symptoms Improve, write a percentage to indicate how much better you feel each week. For example, the first week you feel 15% better, the second week you're 40% better, and so on.

Healing won't happen overnight, so give your body time to heal. You can choose to track your progress in two weeks or ten weeks, depending on how closely you want to reassess your progress. You're in control of the process.

Initially, I recommend checking the Health Graph every four to six weeks. Later, when your health is much better and you're not actively working on something, take the Health Graph every three months to monitor and fine-tune your health.

That's the strength of working with the Health Graph. You are able to evaluate how your body functions at any time and can constantly adapt the support you use to restore your body's optimal function.

Using the Health Graph

1. Graph the Questionnaire results.
2. Pick the highest two or three scores from the list.
3. Follow the suggestions for each area you've chosen to work on.
4. Fill out the Main Symptoms list.
5. Track your progress on the Main Symptoms list.
6. Keep going until you do another Health Questionnaire.
7. Repeat the process until you're perfect!

Health Graph Example

Name: _____   **Date** ___/___/___   **Test #:** ___

Organ/System	Total	%T	10%	20%	30%	40%	50%	60%	70%	80%	90%	100%
Digestion Problems	/21											
Liver/Gall Bladder	/48											
Large Intestine	/18											
Allergies	/21											
Immune System	/15											
Blood Sugar Problems	/66											
Vitamin B Deficiency	/72											
Vitamin G Deficiency	/78											
Fatty Acids Deficiency	/60											
High Autonomic	/42											
Low Autonomic	/39											
High Pituitary	/18											
Low Pituitary	/21											
High Thyroid	/27											
Low Thyroid	/30											
High Adrenal	/15											
Low Adrenal	/48											
Nutritional Deficiency	/78											
Heart Function	/18											
Female Hormonal	/36											
Male Hormonal	/30											

	Main Symptoms	**Percent Symptoms Improve**
1	_____	
2	_____	
3	_____	
4	_____	
5	_____	

OVERVIEW: _____
_____
_____

Health Graph Example

Name: Linda Smith   Date ___/___/___   Test #: __1__

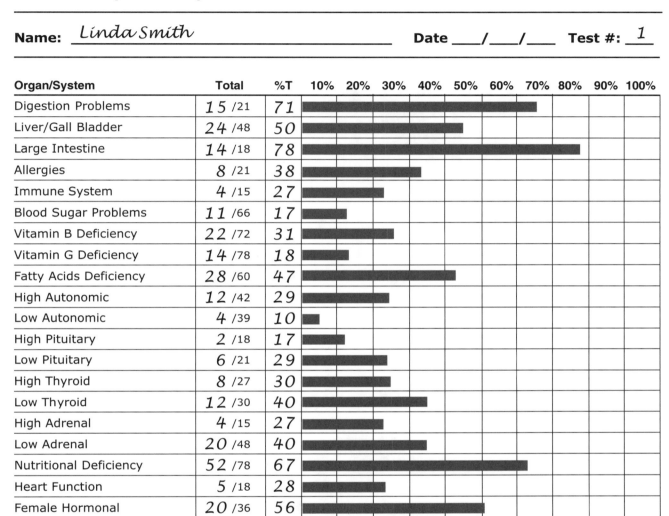

Organ/System	Total	%T	10%	20%	30%	40%	50%	60%	70%	80%	90%	100%
Digestion Problems	15 /21	71										
Liver/Gall Bladder	24 /48	50										
Large Intestine	14 /18	78										
Allergies	8 /21	38										
Immune System	4 /15	27										
Blood Sugar Problems	11 /66	17										
Vitamin B Deficiency	22 /72	31										
Vitamin G Deficiency	14 /78	18										
Fatty Acids Deficiency	28 /60	47										
High Autonomic	12 /42	29										
Low Autonomic	4 /39	10										
High Pituitary	2 /18	17										
Low Pituitary	6 /21	29										
High Thyroid	8 /27	30										
Low Thyroid	12 /30	40										
High Adrenal	4 /15	27										
Low Adrenal	20 /48	40										
Nutritional Deficiency	52 /78	67										
Heart Function	5 /18	28										
Female Hormonal	20 /36	56										
Male Hormonal	0 /30	0										

	Main Symptoms	Percent Symptoms Improve									
1	Gas and bloating	10	25	50	60	70	80				
2	Constipation	20	40	70	90	90	90				
3	Heavy periods	?	?	?	50	?	?				
4	Headaches	15	20	30	50	60	60				
5	Insomnia	0	20	40	40	50	50				

OVERVIEW: Linda's graph reveals her three highest indicators to be <u>Digestion Problems</u>, <u>Large Intestine</u>, and <u>Nutritional Deficiency</u>. <u>Female Hormonal</u> is also high, but is most likely being caused — or made worse — by the other higher-scoring problems. If she chooses to work on <u>Nutritional Deficiency</u>, she should look to that section for interpretation of each symptom.

Health Graph Example

Name: _Linda Smith_   Date ___/___/___   Test #: _2_

Organ/System	Total	%T	10%	20%	30%	40%	50%	60%	70%	80%	90%	100%
Digestion Problems	6 /21	29										
Liver/Gall Bladder	22 /48	46										
Large Intestine	7 /18	38										
Allergies	8 /21	38										
Immune System	3 /15	20										
Blood Sugar Problems	8 /66	12										
Vitamin B Deficiency	18 /72	25										
Vitamin G Deficiency	10 /78	13										
Fatty Acids Deficiency	20 /60	33										
High Autonomic	18 /42	43										
Low Autonomic	3 /39	7										
High Pituitary	2 /18	11										
Low Pituitary	6 /21	29										
High Thyroid	8 /27	30										
Low Thyroid	12 /30	40										
High Adrenal	4 /15	27										
Low Adrenal	14 /48	42										
Nutritional Deficiency	52 /78	67										
Heart Function	5 /18	28										
Female Hormonal	13 /36	36										
Male Hormonal	0 /30	0										

	Main Symptoms	Percent Symptoms Improve									
1	Insomnia	10	25	50	60	70	80				
2	Headaches	20	20	20	40	50	70				
3	Heavy periods	?	?	80	?	?	?				
4	Stiff & Achy	15	20	30	50	70	90				
5	Depression	0	20	40	40	50	60				

OVERVIEW: Linda's second graph shows improvement. The emphasis now is on <u>Liver/Gall Bladder</u> and <u>Nutritional Deficiency</u>. Support <u>Liver/Gall Bladder</u> and take a close look to see what is holding things up in <u>Nutritional Deficiency</u>. The section on <u>Nutritional Deficiency</u> can always be checked for patterns indicating a need for a particular vitamin or mineral.

Health Graph Example

Name: *Mike Miller*   **Date** ___/___/___   **Test #:** ___1___

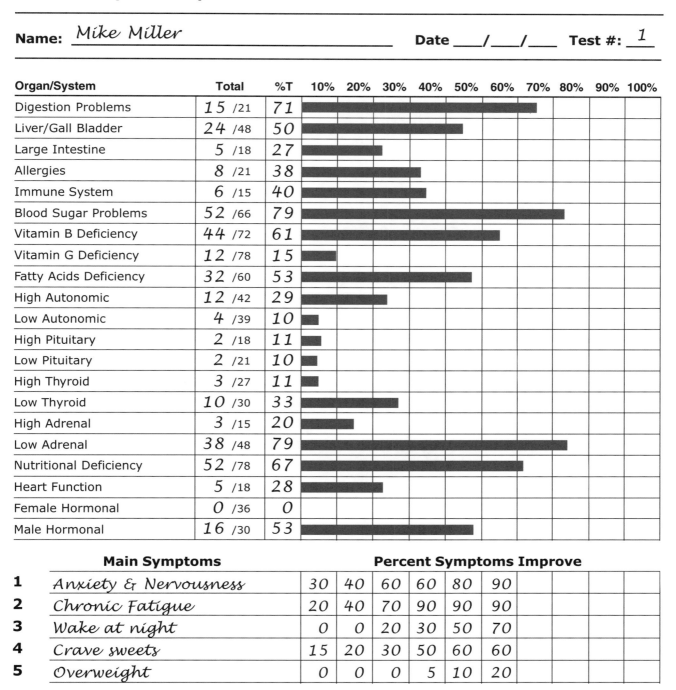

Organ/System	Total	%T
Digestion Problems	15 /21	71
Liver/Gall Bladder	24 /48	50
Large Intestine	5 /18	27
Allergies	8 /21	38
Immune System	6 /15	40
Blood Sugar Problems	52 /66	79
Vitamin B Deficiency	44 /72	61
Vitamin G Deficiency	12 /78	15
Fatty Acids Deficiency	32 /60	53
High Autonomic	12 /42	29
Low Autonomic	4 /39	10
High Pituitary	2 /18	11
Low Pituitary	2 /21	10
High Thyroid	3 /27	11
Low Thyroid	10 /30	33
High Adrenal	3 /15	20
Low Adrenal	38 /48	79
Nutritional Deficiency	52 /78	67
Heart Function	5 /18	28
Female Hormonal	0 /36	0
Male Hormonal	16 /30	53

#	Main Symptoms	Percent Symptoms Improve									
1	Anxiety & Nervousness	30	40	60	60	80	90				
2	Chronic Fatigue	20	40	70	90	90	90				
3	Wake at night	0	0	20	30	50	70				
4	Crave sweets	15	20	30	50	60	60				
5	Overweight	0	0	0	5	10	20				

OVERVIEW: Mike's graph shows several areas of concern that are close in number. The general rule – pick the top two or three to work on – still applies. In this example, it would be <u>Blood Sugar</u> and <u>Digestion Problems</u>. He might also want to include <u>Low Adrenal</u>.

Health Graph Example

Name: _Sherry Mangione_　　　　　**Date** ___/___/___　**Test #:** _1_

Organ/System	Total	%T	10%	20%	30%	40%	50%	60%	70%	80%	90%	100%
Digestion Problems	0 /21	0										
Liver/Gall Bladder	10 /48	21	██									
Large Intestine	4 /18	22	██									
Allergies	5 /21	24	███									
Immune System	2 /15	13	█									
Blood Sugar Problems	45 /66	68	███████									
Vitamin B Deficiency	28 /72	39	████									
Vitamin G Deficiency	14 /78	18	██									
Fatty Acids Deficiency	18 /60	30	███									
High Autonomic	30 /42	71	███████									
Low Autonomic	2 /39	5	█									
High Pituitary	0 /18	0										
Low Pituitary	18 /21	86	█████████									
High Thyroid	2 /27	7	█									
Low Thyroid	23 /30	77	████████									
High Adrenal	2 /15	13	█									
Low Adrenal	39 /48	81	████████									
Nutritional Deficiency	16 /78	21	██									
Heart Function	3 /18	17	██									
Female Hormonal	28 /36	78	████████									
Male Hormonal	0 /30	0										

	Main Symptoms	Percent Symptoms Improve									
1	Fatigue	10	30	30	50	70	90				
2	Irregular Periods	?	?	40	?	?	?				
3	Moodiness	20	30	50	60	80	80				
4	Depression	20	40	50	70	90	95				
5	Can't Concentrate	0	10	30	50	50	60				

OVERVIEW: Sherry's graph shows a common, confusing pattern. Testing high are <u>Low Thyroid</u>, <u>Low Adrenal</u>, and <u>Female Hormonal</u>. Since the pituitary controls all of the glands, start with supporting <u>Low Pituitary</u>. Then focus on <u>Blood Sugar Problems</u> (the cause of a lot of hormonal problems) and <u>Low Pituitary</u>.

Health Graph Example

Name: *David Swanson* **Date** ___/___/___ **Test #:** _1_

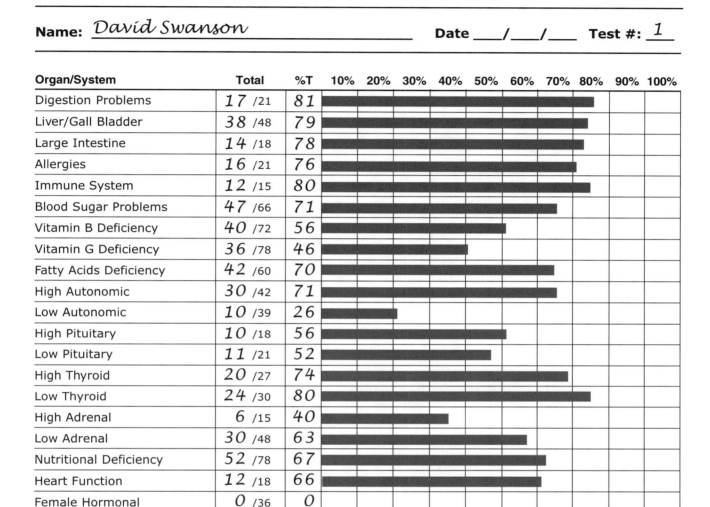

Organ/System	Total	%T	10%	20%	30%	40%	50%	60%	70%	80%	90%	100%
Digestion Problems	17 /21	81										
Liver/Gall Bladder	38 /48	79										
Large Intestine	14 /18	78										
Allergies	16 /21	76										
Immune System	12 /15	80										
Blood Sugar Problems	47 /66	71										
Vitamin B Deficiency	40 /72	56										
Vitamin G Deficiency	36 /78	46										
Fatty Acids Deficiency	42 /60	70										
High Autonomic	30 /42	71										
Low Autonomic	10 /39	26										
High Pituitary	10 /18	56										
Low Pituitary	11 /21	52										
High Thyroid	20 /27	74										
Low Thyroid	24 /30	80										
High Adrenal	6 /15	40										
Low Adrenal	30 /48	63										
Nutritional Deficiency	52 /78	67										
Heart Function	12 /18	66										
Female Hormonal	0 /36	0										
Male Hormonal	24 /30	80										

	Main Symptoms	Percent Symptoms Improve									
1	*Fatigue*	10	25	50	60	70	80				
2	*Muscle & joint pain*	20	40	70	90	90	90				
3	*Headaches*	10	10	30	40	70	80				
4	*Foggy-headed*	15	20	30	50	60	70				
5	*Anxiety*	0	20	40	40	50	60				

OVERVIEW: Although David's graph involves many areas, this is a good example of a need to focus on digestion. Look to the sections on <u>Digestion Problems</u>, <u>Liver/Gall Bladder</u>, and <u>Large Intestine</u>. If available, your most recent lab results may help you determine the area(s) under the most stress. Consider a cleanse from <u>The Elements of Health: Detoxification and Fasting</u>. These issues often clear up on follow-up health graphs.

Interpreting the Results

Refer to How To Use The Workbook: Workbook Vocabulary and Definitions for interpretation of the recommendations in this section.

Digestion Problems

Both your stomach and pancreas, lying immediately below your rib cage on the left side, release digestive enzymes that control the breakdown and absorption of your food. Digestive enzymes also regulate the pH of the intestines, create the proper environment for healthy bacteria in your gut, protect you from infection, and regulate the peristalsis (muscular action) of your intestines for proper elimination.

In general, you need to eat more whole food (and less junk food). See the recommendations found in The Elements of Health: Foundation Diet for more information. Drinking more water will make a huge difference in your digestion.

Digestion Problems are often caused by deficiencies of zinc, B vitamins, and salt. Check for a zinc deficiency under Nutritional Deficiency in this section and with Using Home Tests: The Zinc Taste Test. Also, check the sections for Vitamin B Deficiency and Vitamin G Deficiency in the Health Graph, because the B vitamin complex is needed to make digestive enzymes. Salt (as in Celtic salt) is also a necessary nutrient.

Unless your digestion works correctly, it's pretty difficult to be healthy. Many hormone problems, allergies, chronic fatigue, anemia, and mineral deficiencies (like calcium and iron) are due to poor digestion. One theory purports that aging is due to chronic malnutrition from digestive problems. People who suffer from chronic fatigue syndrome, fibromyalgia syndrome, osteoarthritis, rheumatoid arthritis, and many other problems usually find remarkable relief once they get their digestion sorted out.

Digestive problems are usually due to a lack of stomach enzymes (hydrochloric acid), pancreatic enzymes, or both.

You'll know when your digestion is right because you won't notice it! You won't experience gas, bloating, indigestion, constipation, or the myriad of other things that go along with bad digestion.

To correct Digestive Problems, refer to the Digestive Dysfunction chart. Many companies make digestive enzymes and many good digestive enzymes are available, but in my opinion, Biotics makes the best of the best.

Primary Support: General Digestive Enzyme Formula
   *** Source: Hydrozyme (BRC) 1-6 tablets with meals
    ** Source: Digestive Enzymes (generic) as directed

Start with a general formula to support digestion controlled by both the stomach and pancreas. Hydrozyme, a formula including both stomach and pancreatic enzymes, will generally make a big difference in your digestion. Sometimes, though, you need to use very specific combinations of enzymes, as the Digestive Dysfunction chart below shows. If you find that using a general combination formula doesn't help you after a week or two, work through the Digestive Dysfunction chart.

Start with one tablet or capsule per meal and then increase by one tablet or capsule per meal every one or two days. When you get to the right dosage, you will notice the symptoms related to your digestion will clear. Take enough of the digestive enzymes so there is no gas, bloating, or indigestion, and your bowel movements are regular.

If you notice cramping or burning sensations that are relieved when you eat, decrease your dosage slightly. Using these guidelines will allow you to adjust the dosage to your needs. In most cases, the dosage will be relatively high initially (4-6 tabs/caps per meal), but will decrease over time (1-2/meal).

The need for supplementary digestive enzymes may be temporary. As your health improves, you may be able to produce enough digestive enzymes on your own. If you're more than 50 years of age, you will probably need to continue taking some kind of digestive enzyme for optimum health. Take the time and effort it may take to work through digestive problems. Your health won't get better, no matter what else you do, until any problems with digestion are resolved.

Digestive Dysfunction

Symptoms include gas, bloating, indigestion, bad breath, loss of taste for meat, difficulty digesting raw food, and constipation.

Stomach Dysfunction	Pancreas Dysfunction
• Loss of taste for meat • Belching shortly after eating • Indigestion ¼-1 hour after eating	• Indigestion 1-2 hours after eating • Problems digesting raw food • Undigested food in stool
Try: • HCl Plus (BRC)	**Try:** • Bromelain PlusCLA (BRC)
Without improvement, try instead: • Betaine Plus (BRC)	**Without improvement, try instead:** • Intenzyme Forte (BRC)
Without improvement, try instead: • Hydrozyme (BRC)	**Without improvement, try instead:** • Bio-6 Plus (BRC)
Without improvement, consult a physician practicing functional medicine.	**Without improvement, try instead:** • Hydrozyme (BRC)
	Without improvement, consult a physician practicing functional medicine.

Determining Dosage

Start with 1 tablet/capsule per meal and increase by 1 tablet/capsule per meal every 1-2 days until all symptoms are clear. If you begin to experience stomach burning that is relieved by eating, decrease the dosage slightly until the burning is gone.

HCL Plus, Betaine Plus, and Bromelain-PlusCLA are vegetarian sources of enzymes. Intenzyme Forte, Bio-6 Plus, and Hydrozyme are not vegetarian formulas.

Liver/Gall Bladder

Your liver and gall bladder lie just below your ribs on the right side.

Your liver is one of the most complex organs in your body. It's responsible for balancing your blood sugar, maintaining the balance of amino acids in your body, detoxifying harmful chemicals you're exposed to in your environment as well as those you make within your body as a normal part of metabolism, producing cholesterol and triglycerides for storage of energy and to make hormones, making bile for the elimination of excess cholesterol, digesting fat-soluble nutrients, and activating and deactivating hormones.

The gall bladder stores bile where it is available as needed for proper digestion of fats and fat-soluble nutrients. Bile also circulates cholesterol into your intestinal tract for elimination, stimulates peristalsis (the muscular action of the intestines), and balances the flora in the intestinal tract.

Congestion in the liver and gall bladder (including the bile ducts) is an extremely common problem, and no wonder. You're constantly exposed to a huge list of chemicals in your environment that you were never designed to handle. Solvents, plastics, pesticides, formaldehyde, flavorings, colorings, preservatives, lead, mercury, aluminum, copper pipes, gasoline, air pollutants — they're all toxic to your body.

Your liver may be overwhelmed trying to filter your system of all these toxic chemicals and may not be able to keep up with all the other things it's in charge of, such as helping the rest of your body make protein, balancing blood sugar, controlling cholesterol and blood pressure, and activating and deactivating hormones.

One way to tell if you have a gall bladder or bile duct problem is if fatty, fried foods and/or raw garlic or onions cause you indigestion. Gall bladders weren't designed to handle margarine or other hydrogenated fats, white flour (or anything made with it), or sugar. All these foods clog up the gall bladder and bile ducts. Avoid them as much as possible.

Primary Support:	Bile Thinning Agents
*** Source:	Beta TCP (BRC): 1-2 tablets TID with meals
** Source:	Lecithin (generic/BRC): 2 capsules/perles with each meal or 3 capsules BID
Note:	Biotics lecithin is labeled Phosphatidylcholine
Secondary Support:	Herbal Liver Support
*** Source:	Livotrit (BRC): 1-2 tablets with each meal
** Source:	Generic Burdock Root: 10-40 drops of tincture after each meal

Consider doing a cleanse from The Elements of Health: Detoxification and Fasting.

Large Intestine

The most common problem here is dysbiosis, meaning you don't have the right kind of bacteria in your gut. Maintaining an ideal balance of bacteria in your gut makes a profound difference in your health. Many people in the healing arts are convinced that disease and premature aging result from abnormal flora and toxicity in the large intestine.

Primary Support:	Bulk and General Support Formula
*** Source:	Colon-Plus (BRC): 1-6 capsules BID with lots of water
** Source:	Psyllium Hulls (generic): 1-6 capsules BID or 1 tsp–1 Tbsp with lots of water
Secondary Support:	Acidophilis Formula
*** Source:	Biodophilis-FOS (BRC): ½–2 tsps a day
** Source:	Acidophilis Formula (generic): as directed

Most people don't get enough fiber in their diet. Taking a source of fiber like the Colon Plus or Psyllium Hulls is useful. The Colon Plus Powder is a fantastic product having psyllium, flax, acidophilus, digestive enzymes, and a few other things for good measure. Taking the primary and secondary support together can make huge improvements in your gut function. Be sure to drink more water and eat more whole foods, especially vegetables. Consider a cleanse from The Elements of Health: Detoxification and Fasting.

Allergies

Most people associate allergies with hay fever that manifests as itchy and watery eyes, lung and nasal congestion, and chronic sinus problems or reactions to foods that include hives and throat itching and swelling. These are the immediate type (IgE-mediated) allergic reactions.

The delayed (IgG-mediated) reactions are more insidious. Typical delayed allergic reactions are fatigue, joint and muscle stiffness and pain, headaches, feeling foggy-headed, anxiety, poor sleep, waking up tired in the morning, and weight gain.

In fact, weight gain is so common with delayed allergic reactions that anyone who has trouble losing weight despite eating less, and who has increased their intake of whole foods and is exercising more, should be tested for food allergies.

Dealing with allergies first requires clearing up Digestion Problems, Liver/Gall Bladder, Large Intestine, and High Adrenal or Low Adrenal. Eat more whole foods and drink plenty of water. Allergies often are related to chronic dehydration. Decreasing exposure to chemicals in your environment (solvents, pesticides, etc.) will help tremendously.

Primary Support:	Histidine
*** Source:	Generic/BRC Histidine: 1-2 tabs BID or TID
Secondary Support:	pH Balance
*** Source:	Bio-CMP (BRC): 2 tabs TID
** Source:	Miixed Ascorbate Powder (BRC): 1 heaping tsp BID or TID
Tertiary Support:	Una de Gato
*** Source:	Una de Gato (AHC): 1-2D BID/TID or 1-2 caps BID/TID

As acid-alkaline balance is critical to resolving allergy, refer to Body pH in the Home Test section. Apple cider vinegar is particularly useful.

For practical purposes, the most common allergies are associated with the following foods in (roughly) their order of frequency:

- Milk and milk products, including cheese (butter is usually okay)
- Wheat and other grains
- Citrus foods (oranges, grapefruit, lemon, lime)
- Nightshade-related foods (tomatoes, potatoes, peppers, eggplant)
- Yeast and molds (cultured foods like cheese, breads, yogurt, etc.)
- Soy

You can often determine which foods give you trouble by avoiding all of them for a couple of weeks and then introducing them one at a time to see how you react. Keep a journal to track symptoms. Introduce only one type of food every two to three days, because it may take that long for the related symptoms to appear.

Immune System

Your immune system is comprised of the thymus, spleen, adrenal glands, and lymph nodes. This system is your defense against infection. It aids in the repair of injuries and regulates your response to allergens.

Your thymus, found just behind the notch found at the top of your sternum, controls your immediate immune response.

Your spleen, found beneath your stomach and ribs on your left side, controls long-term resistance and immune response and also plays a role in regulating red blood cells.

Your adrenals are tiny glands found immediately above each kidney. Always check High Adrenal and Low Adrenal when problems with Immune System or Allergies are present. Adrenal Dysfunction is probably the most common cause of Allergies and Immune System dysfunction.

If your immune system is weak, you'll be prone to getting infections and they will tend to hang on far too long. If your immune system is poorly regulated (usually in response to chronic stress), you will be prone to allergies and autoimmune diseases like rheumatoid arthritis, multiple sclerosis, and lupus.

Primary Support:	Broad Scope Nutritional, Glandular and Herbal Immune Formula
*** Source:	Bio-Immunozyme (BRC): 1-2 tabs BID or TID for 1-3 months; long-term support at 1-2 tabs a day
Secondary Support:	Arabinogalactins
*** Source:	IAG 1-2 (BRC): 1-2 tsp TID for 1-3 months; long-term support at 1-2 tsp a day
Teriary Support:	Una de Gato
*** Source:	Una de Gato (AHC): 1-2 D TID
** Source:	Una de Gato (generic): 1-2 D TID (*Note:* A distant second to AHC)

Blood Sugar Problems

Your liver, adrenal glands, and pancreas work as a team to regulate your blood sugar. Problems with blood sugar mean your body doesn't have the fuel it needs for energy, or that it has too much fuel that can't be burned properly, predisposing you to diabetes and heart disease.

Cortisol, a hormone from the adrenal glands, stimulates your liver to turn fat and proteins into sugar, and then into energy, in every cell in your body. Your pancreas controls your blood sugar with two hormones: glucagon (which raises your blood sugar) and insulin (which lowers your blood sugar).

Blood sugar problems can be caused or aggravated by Digestion Problems, Liver/Gall Bladder, Allergies, and Low Adrenal. Look to these sections for a possible solution to blood sugar problems.

Too much sugar (carbohydrates) in your diet is the most likely cause of blood sugar problems. Excess carbohydrates come from over-consumption of breads, pasta, pizza, sodas, ice cream, candies, pastries, and juices. Most foods labeled low-fat are too high in sugar.

For your diet, use the guidelines from The Elements of Health: Foundation Diet and decrease or eliminate your consumption of grains, a lot of fruit, and fruit juices. Eat more often so your blood sugar stays level. Vegetarians are often guilty of eating too many carbohydrates (starches and sugars). If you're a vegetarian, make sure to focus on protein-rich foods and vegetables.

Primary Support:	B Vitamin, Trace Mineral and Amino Acid Formula
*** Source:	Nutritional Yeast (KAL) 2 Tbsp BID
** Source:	Bio-Glycozyme (BRC): 1-2 tablets BID or TID; 10am, 3pm, 9pm
* Source:	KAL Nutritional Yeast Tablets (KAL): 4-8 tablets BID or TID
Secondary Support:	Insulin-Regulating Herbal Formula
*** Source:	Metabazon (AHC): 1-2 D BID/TID or 1-2 caps BID/TID
Tertiary Support:	Soy Protein
***Source:	Gamoctapro (BRC): 1-2 servings a day
**Source:	Generic Soy Protein: 1-2 servings a day

Vitamin B Deficiency and Vitamin G Deficiency

Eating junk and packaged food and drinking sodas and coffee deplete your body of B vitamins necessary for your body to make energy. It's no wonder many people feel tired most of the time.

To get more B vitamins in your diet, eat more whole and unprocessed foods. You can't get B vitamins from taking the typical B vitamin supplements. High-potency B vitamins (25 mg, or even 100 mg of each B vitamin) are mostly useless and can even cause you problems such as stress on your liver and mineral depletion. Real B vitamins, usually labeled phosphorylated, contain phosphorus.

All high-potency B vitamin formulas must be activated (phosphorylated) in your liver before they can function in your body. Often your liver can't do this because it's too busy detoxifying environmental toxins or doesn't have available the necessary nutrients.

The B vitamin complex is composed of the water-soluble fraction known as Vitamin B, and the alcohol-soluble fraction is known as Vitamin G. They have different functions, and being able to determine the exact fraction needed can be very useful. G and B complexes together are very important to enzyme reactions and making energy.

Here is a breakdown of the Vitamin B and Vitamin G fractions:

B Vitamin Complex	
Vitamin B **(Water-soluble)** *Consists primarily of:* Thiamine (B1) Cobalamin (B12) Pantothenic Acid (B5)	**Vitamin G** **(Alcohol-soluble)** *Consists primarily of:* Niacin (B2) Riboflavin (B3) Folic Acid, Choline, and Inositol

Interpreting B & G Deficiency Syndrome

Results	What to Do		
Primary B Vitamin Deficiency	Bio-3BG	(BRC)	6 tabs TID for 1B 6 tabs BID for 1B 3 tabs BID for 1B 1-3 tabs a day as needed
Primary G Vitamin Deficiency	Bio-GGGB	(BRC)	6 tabs TID for 1B 6 tabs BID for 1B 3 tabs BID for 1B 1-3 tabs a day as needed
B Complex Deficiency	Nutritional Yeast Bio-B 100	(KAL) (BRC)	2 Tablespoons BID 6 tabs TID for 1B 6 tabs BID for 1B 3 tabs BID for 1B 1-3 tabs a day as needed

High score on Vitamin B deficiency = primary Vitamin B deficiency
High score on Vitamin G deficiency = primary Vitamin G deficiency
High score for both B and G = B-complex deficiency
Chewing supplements will increase their effectiveness.
1B = 1 bottle

This heavy dosage makes a significant difference in a short time. Since I began recommending this accelerated dosage, people notice big changes in a week rather than a month. There is no harm in taking these high dosages, because B-complex vitamins are water-soluble or alcohol-soluble and don't build up in your system like fat-soluble nutrients do.

It's likely you'll look at the dosage on the label of these natural, food-based vitamins and wonder what you're paying for, since the dosage per tablet is much lower than high-potency B vitamin supplements. The high-potency B vitamins, however, don't equate to those in a natural form.

I commonly see people in my practice taking 100 mg per day of high-potency B vitamin complex and still suffering from B vitamin deficiency, both in their lab findings and in the symptoms. When they begin taking 3-18 mg per day of the low-potency B vitamins in a natural form, they get better.

Occasionally, I recommend using wheat germ as a strategy to clear up a B vitamin complex deficiency, either alone or in combination with supplementation. Although fresh wheat germ is in theory the best form, it goes rancid very rapidly. I recommend getting wheat germ from the grocery store and eating ½-1 cup a day. Keep it in the refrigerator, or better yet, in the freezer once the bottle is opened so the wheat germ won't go rancid.

Wheat germ has a very pleasant flavor. Many people enjoy eating it directly, though some blend it with juice or a smoothie or mix it in yogurt. Wheat germ, along with nutritional yeast, often helps when nothing else has worked. Just be aware that it is wheat; avoid it if you have a wheat allergy.

Fatty Acids Deficiency

Essential fatty acids regulate your body chemistry at every level. Deficiency of essential fatty acids is extremely common for three reasons: food-refining removes the naturally occurring essential fatty acids from whole foods, low-fat diets are deficient in natural fats and oils, and the amount of hydrogenated fats that are present in packaged foods.

Hydrogenated fats (including margarine) aren't healthy for you. Hydrogenated fats block the normal actions of essential fatty acids and cause increased blood clotting (predisposing you to heart attack and strokes), increase inflammation (causing pain), and impair the normal metabolism of hormones throughout your body (causing male and female hormonal problems).

Using Home Tests: Body pH will confirm a need for essential fatty acids and help you monitor your improvement as you change your diet and use supplemental oils.

Interpreting the Essential Fatty Acid Need		
Score	**Meaning**	**What to Do**
0-20%	No deficiency	Nothing
21-35%	Mild deficiency	• Flax Oil (generic/BRC) 2-4 capsules a day after a meal. • Use the Foundation Diet. • Avoid hydrogenated oils (especially margarine!).
36-49%	Moderate deficiency	• Flax Oil (generic/BRC) 2-4 capsules TID after meals. • Use the Foundation Diet. • Avoid hydrogenated oils (especially margarine!).
50-100%	Marked deficiency	• Flax Oil (generic) 1-2 Tablespoons BID or TID with or after meals. • Use the Foundation Diet. • Avoid hydrogenated oils (especially margarine!).

For all of my patients, I recommend a pleasant tasting, cinnamon-flavored flax oil made by Spectrum.

Essential fatty-acid deficiency is a huge issue and has a profound impact on your health. It has been estimated that primitive diets have about six times the levels of essential fatty acids of modern "civilized" diets. Eating whole foods according to the Foundation Diet will naturally tend to clear up essential fatty-acid deficiencies (The Elements of Health: Foundation Diet).

Autonomic Nervous System

The very first thing I address when people come to see me is the balance of their autonomic nervous system. Since it regulates every part of the body, I know that if I don't get this system back in balance, they won't get better — no matter what else I do.

The autonomic nervous system regulates every unconscious process in your body. Think of it as the *automatic* part of your nervous system. It has to be set properly for the systems of your body to function optimally and in harmony.

There are two parts to the autonomic nervous system:

- **Parasympathetic** — It's like the brakes: it slows you down, relaxes you, and controls all your body functions so they can work together in a relaxed state.

- **Sympathetic** — It's like the gas pedal: it speeds you up and controls everything to do with the flight-or-fight response.

Your body needs to function primarily in a parasympathetic state, because that's when your body repairs and maintains itself. If your body stays in a sympathetic (fight-or-flight) state for extended periods of the time, it will break down faster than it can repair itself.

High Autonomic (Sympathetic Dominant)

A High Autonomic (Sympathetic Dominant) state is one of the most harmful health problems you can have. That's because the effects are so damaging, so insidious, so far-reaching, and so often misdiagnosed.

When your body is in a High Autonomic state, it breaks down from stress. Symptoms can show up in a variety of ways. High Autonomic states will always create High Adrenal initially and Low Adrenal eventually. To really understand the implications of this health problem, I recommend reading the section titled Stress and Life.

Low Autonomic (Parasympathetic Dominant)

Long-term effects of this health problem are tendencies to developing diabetes, cardiovascular disease, and Low Thyroid. The Parasympathetic Dominant state also predisposes you to osteoarthritis, bursitis, calcific tendonitis, and gall bladder disease.

The most obvious and immediate problem with being Parasympathetic Dominant has to do with energy and drive. Being Parasympathetic Dominant will make a person feel lackadaisical and without drive and energy. Balancing the Parasympathetic Dominant state increases energy, mental clarity, and focus.

Interpreting The Autonomic Nervous System

Score	Meaning	What to Do
High Autonomic >20%	Mild	Parasympa (DR): 1-2 D BID Alternate-Nostril Breathing
High Autonomic >40%	Moderate	Parasympa (DR): 2 D TID Alternate-Nostril Breathing Bio GGGB (BRC): 3-6 tabs TID
High Autonomic >60%	Severe	Parasympa (DR): 2 D TID Alternate-Nostril Breathing Bio GGGB (BRC): 3-6 tabs TID Bio-CMP (BRC): 4 tabs TID
Low Autonomic >20%	Mild	Bio-3BG (BRC): 3 tabs BID
Low Autonomic >40%	Moderate	Lecithin (generic/BRC): 2-3 BID Bio-3BG (BRC): 4 tabs TID
Low Autonomic >60%	Severe	Liquid Phosphozyme (BRC): 1-2 D BID Lecithin (generic/BRC): 2-3 BID Bio-3BG (BRC): 4 tabs TID

> greater than

Alternate-Nostril Breathing is covered in The Elements of Health: Contemplation, Meditation and Prayer.

On Parasympa

Parasympa is an herbal tincture (liquid extract) made of damiana, kava, and oat seed. The oat seed, collected when still green, releases a rich milky liquid when squeezed between your fingers. These herbs are traditionally used to help people with nervous exhaustion, or, as it's referred to these days, chronic fatigue syndrome. Parasympa increases the tone of the parasympathetic nervous system. It helps people relax. I consider it the first stage of getting someone well when they are unable to relax or suffer from chronic stress.

It's interesting to note that these herbs are reputed to be aphrodisiacs. Sexual response is controlled mostly by the Parasympathetic nervous system. If you're in a High Autonomic (Sympathetic Dominant) state, it's very difficult to get in the mood sexually. If your body is stuck in a fight-or-flight response, it doesn't consider sex to be a high priority. It's not important for immediate survival. The reason your body can't respond is because the circuit for getting turned on is shut off. Getting your autonomic nervous system balanced opens up that circuit and your body can respond sexually.

You may feel very tired for the first 3-7 days. The more you've depleted your body from stress, the longer and more profoundly you will feel tired. After that, your energy will build, but it will be relaxed, real energy. You will know you're on the right track when after a few days you start to feel more rested when you wake up.

Often with very chronic stress and over-stimulation, you experience nervous exhaustion. Any time there has been severe and/or chronic stress in your life and you experience fatigue or even exhaustion, take Parasympa. It is the most consistently useful remedy for stress I have ever used. I usually have people take two droppers-full in water three times a day for six weeks. Then take Parasympa afterwards as needed.

Some people end up doing very well by taking a little bit of Parasympa on a regular basis. The dosage is best regulated in the long run based on how you feel. You will ideally feel relaxed and more energetic. You will also be able to handle stressful situations more easily. The ongoing need for this remedy is usually due to either being under ongoing stress or because of a genetic tendency to being <u>High Autonomic</u> (Sympathetic Dominant).

Pituitary

Your pituitary rests between the hemispheres of your brain and behind your eyes. It regulates your thyroid, maintains bone density and muscle mass, and controls metabolism (including blood sugar balance and body repair), male and female hormone levels, adrenal glands, and blood pressure.

High Pituitary

The Type A person is always pushing, can never relax, and looks at sleep as a waste of time. If you fit that picture, you probably experience a crash once in a while. After getting some extra rest, you'll be up and running until the next crash. As you get older, the crashes get to be more and more often, and they last longer.

It's better to calm down your pituitary. Once you do, you'll feel more relaxed with more even and dependable energy.

Primary Support:	Pituitary Gland
***Source:	Cytozyme PT/HPT (BRC): 1-2 tablets BID or TID; chew
Secondary Support:	Damiana and Oats Formula
***Source:	Parasympa (DR) 1-2 D BID or TID
**Source:	You can mix equal parts of damiana and oats (milky oat seed) using tinctures (alcohol-soluble herbal extracts) from health food stores; 1-2 D BID or TID

You might feel pretty tired and sleepy when you first start this program. Don't worry! That means it's doing exactly what it's supposed to do. Your energy will return after a few days and it will be calmer and deeper.

Trace mineral deficiencies can cause pituitary imbalances. Eat a whole-food diet and take a good multiple-vitamin/mineral supplement. Make sure that the multiple you take has no iron or copper unless you're anemic. Feeling hyped up, anxious, and unable to relax is often due to having too little zinc and too much copper in your body. Check <u>Nutritional Deficiency</u> in this section and the <u>Zinc Taste Test</u> (<u>Using Home Tests: The Zinc Taste Test</u>) for a zinc deficiency.

Low Pituitary
The pituitary regulates the thyroid and adrenal glands, male and female hormone levels, blood sugar, rate of healing, and fluid regulation. Look to the pituitary as a likely culprit when there are imbalances of multiple body systems or when treatment to any of these areas produces only temporary, limited, or non-existent results.

Primary Support:	Gamma-Oryzanol
***Source:	Gammanol forte (BRC): 1-2 tablets BID or TID; chew
Secondary Support:	Maca Root
***Source:	Sumacazon (RBE): 1-2 capsules or 1-2 D BID or TID
**Source:	B-Vital (BRC): 1-2 capsules BID
*Source:	Generic Maca: 2-4 capsules BID or TID

Make sure you get lots of good-quality protein in your diet. Your pituitary is very sensitive to insufficient protein.

Manganese, a trace mineral, is as important to your pituitary as iodine is to your thyroid. Consider supplementing with manganese (Mn-Zyme Forte (BRC; 1-3 tabs per day)) if you don't see improvement with the above regimen.

Thyroid

Your thyroid is found below your Adam's apple and above your sternum. Its primary function is to stimulate your metabolism, and its secondary function is to stimulate your immune system.

High Thyroid
With High Thyroid you will be tense, anxious, and tired. Interestingly, anxious exhaustion is probably the most consistent symptom of high thyroid. Stress is the most common cause of high thyroid. Check for High Autonomic. Simplify your life, sleep more, eat well, find a passion in your life that fulfills you, and have more fun.

Primary Support:	Natural Lithium (Essential Trace Mineral)
*** Source:	LI-Zyme Forte (BRC): 1 tablet TID
Secondary Support:	Vitamin A
*** Source:	Bio-AE Mulsion Forte (BRC): 2-4 d TID
** Source:	Generic Vitamin A 50,000 IU a day (preferably from lemon grass)
Tertiary Support:	Alkaline Minerals
*** Source:	Generic Alfalfa: 3-6 tablets BID
** Source:	K-Zyme (BRC): 2 tablets BID

Low Thyroid

Low thyroid is one of the most misdiagnosed illnesses. It's common for people to have a low thyroid when the lab tests don't show it.

Fluoride and chlorine look like iodine to your body. They compete for the same slots that iodine normally fills. Drinking fluoridated and chlorinated tap water can cause low thyroid. Drink and cook with tap water as little as possible. Bottled water really is better for you, and the best-of-the-best is distilled.

Eat natural oils (olive, sesame, etc.) and fats (cheese, butter, etc.) and stay away from margarine and foods with hydrogenated oils.

Eating a diet high in protein and fats and low in carbohydrates helps to rev up your thyroid. See Using Lab Tests: Blood Fats. Eat more fish and sea vegetables (kelp, dulse, nori, etc.). Check Using Home Tests: Body Temperature and Using Lab Tests: Thyroid.

Have lab work for the tests mentioned in the thyroid done every three months at first to see if you're getting better and make sure you're not over-stimulating your thyroid. If you see your temperature goes above normal, start to score high in High Thyroid, or see your thyroid tests from your lab work go above normal, decrease the thyroid support you're taking so that you're testing in the optimum range.

Primary Support: Thyroid Formula
*** Source: GTA Forte (BRC): 1 capsule BID or TID with meals; if you feel over-stimulated (like drinking too much coffee) when taking GTA, decrease the dosage.

Secondary Support: Thyroid Specific Nutrition
*** Source: Thyrostim (BRC): 1-2 tablets BID or TID with meals

Tertiary Support: Iodine
*** Source: Liquid Iodine (BRC): 4-10 d a day

Adrenal Glands

Your adrenal glands, residing immediately above your kidneys, affect every cell and every function of your body. Because of their importance to your health in general, adrenal glands are covered more completely in Stress and Life.

High Adrenal

This is the person with a short fuse, who's always worried or worked up about something, and who can't relax. Stress is the cause. Make sure to simplify your life, have more fun, rest more, and worry less. Take better care of yourself.

Primary Support: Damiana, Kava & Oats Formula
*** Source: Parasympa (DR): 2 D BID or TID
** Source: Generic mix of the two herbs in a tincture form

Secondary Support: Adrenal Vitamin, Mineral and Herbal Formula
*** Source: ADHS (BRC): 1-2 tabs BID in the morning and afternoon

Tertiary Support: Pituitary Gland
*** Source: Cytozyme PT/HPT (BRC): 1-2 tablets BID or TID; chew

Low Adrenal

This problem wears many masks and mimics many different illnesses. A more complete list can be found in Stress and Life.

Low Adrenal is often the cause underlying allergies, arthritis, hypoglycemia, chronic fatigue, joint and muscle pains, and any immune problem.

Use The Elements of Health strategies as recommended in the previous section for High Adrenal. Balance your blood sugar by eating more whole foods, raw veggies, less sugar and white flour, and more protein. Eat more often and stay away from sodas. Coffee and alcohol should generally be avoided, although small amounts may be tolerated.

Primary Support:	Herbal Adrenal Tonic
*** Source:	Sumacazon (AHC): 1-2 D BID or TID
** Source:	ADHS (BRC): 1-2 tablets in the morning and afternoon
* Source:	Generic American or Siberian Ginseng
Secondary Support:	Adrenal Gland
*** Source:	Cytozyme AD (BRC): 1-2 tablets TID; chewed

Resolving Low Adrenal can be a complicated process. If your adrenal function doesn't respond to the above program, refer to Stress and Life for more strategies on restoring adrenal function.

Nutritional Deficiency

Dietary Intake

With nutritional deficiency, always refer to Using Foods To Balance Body Function to know which foods to increase in your diet.

Absorption

Beside an inadequate diet, poor absorption of food in the small intestines is often the cause of nutritional deficiency. The solution is to use bentonite for a few weeks so you'll be able to get all of the nutrients out of your food more efficiently.

There is an interesting symptom associated with this problem which very consistently indicates the need for bentonite. If you often feel hungry but can't decide what it is you want to eat when you go to the fridge or the cupboard, you need bentonite.

Bentonite is a fine clay that scours the debris (from refined foods lacking fiber) coating the villi of your small intestine. Eliminating this coating from your small intestines exposes the full surface area of your intestines, and dramatically improves digestion and absorption.

Once you've used the bentonite for a few weeks, you will find that you know exactly what you want to eat most of the time. You will also notice clearly and quickly the effects of what you eat, both good and bad, on your body.

Use Cholacol II (SPL) at 4 tablets 15 minutes before meals or Hydrated Bentonite (YP) 1-2 Tbsp in diluted juice for 2-6 weeks. If you're using the Hydrated Bentonite, start with 1 tsp BID and work up to 2 Tbsp BID over 4-10 days. Starting with the full dosage can cause constipation. The Hydrated Bentonite can be mixed in with the Colon Plus Powder. Take these separately from other supplements.

Calcium Deficiency

Frequent Skin Rashes and/or Hives

Take a calcium supplement, ideally with some complementary magnesium. If you do not respond within two days to the supplementation with calcium/magnesium combination, you probably need to include essential fatty acids.

Primary Support:	Calcium/Magnesium Combination
***Source:	Ca/Mg-Zyme (BRC): 1-2 tablets TID
**Source:	Generic Calcium/Magnesium supplement
Note:	If you find the calcium/magnesium combination doesn't work, you may need an acidic calcium source: Bio-CMP (BRC): 1-2 tablets TID
Secondary Support:	Essential Fatty Acids
***Source:	Mixed EFAs (BRC): 1 tsp-2 Tbsp a day as needed to clear symptoms
**Source:	Flax Oil (Spectrum): 1 tsp-2 Tbsp a day or 4-12 capsules/perles a day as needed to clear symptoms

Muscle Cramping of Leg or Foot When at Rest or Sleeping

This is usually a calcium deficiency. If you don't get relief with calcium, add the essential fatty acids as a synergist to get the job done.

Primary Support:	Acid Calcium/ Magnesium Combination
***Source:	Bio-CMP (BRC): 1–2 tablets TID
**Source:	Generic Calcium/Magnesium supplement
Note:	Bio-CMP, an acidic form of calcium, is more bioavailable than regular calcium.
Secondary Support:	Essential Fatty Acids
***Source:	Mixed EFAs (BRC): 1 tsp–2 Tbsp a day as needed to clear symptoms
**Source:	Flax Oil: 1 tsp–2 Tbsp (Spectrum, preferably cinnamon-flavored) a day or 4-12 capsules/perles (generic/BRC) a day as needed to clear symptoms.

Fevers Easily Raised or Frequent

This is either a calcium need or an immune deficiency. If this is not associated with frequent infections, use calcium (same sources and doses as noted previously). If you suffer from frequent infections, get some general immune support:

Primary Support:	General Immune Stimulant Formula
***Source:	Bio-Immunozyme (BRC): 1-2 tablets TID
**Source:	Una de Gato (AHC): 1-2 D TID
* Source:	Generic maitake, astragalus, or shitake mushroom capsules or tinctures or a combination of them.

Magnesium Deficiency

Crave Chocolate

Craving chocolate is nearly always a magnesium deficiency. This is especially true in women who have an overwhelming chocolate craving just before the onset of menstruation.

Primary Support: Magnesium
***Source: Mg-Zyme (BRC) 1-6 tablets before bed
**Source: Generic Magnesium supplement

Note: Start the MG Zyme at 1-2 tablets before bed and increase by one tablet each succeeding night. When you get to the point where you have a loose bowel movement in the morning, decrease the dosage by one tablet. That is your ideal dosage.

Feet Have Bad Odor

This is also a magnesium deficiency. Isn't it nice to have a solution for this problem! Use magnesium as noted previously.

If the magnesium doesn't clear up the problem, check your <u>Digestion Problems</u> and <u>Large Intestine</u>.

Vitamin D Deficiency or Parathyroid Dysfunction

Hoarseness Frequent

This problem develops when your parathyroid glands (the small glands next to your thyroid) don't properly regulate your calcium levels.

Primary Support: Parathyroid Extract
***Source: Ca/Mg-Plus (BRC): 1 tablet BID or TID

Secondary Support: Vitamin D
***Source: Get more natural oils in your diet. Avoid hydrogenated oils. See <u>The Elements of Health: Foundation Diet</u> and get more sun.
Doing these things will help you make your own vitamin D.
**Source: Bio-D-Mulsion (BRC): 1-2 d a day

Potassium Deficiency

Difficulty Swallowing

This can also be a parathyroid problem, though it is more often a need for more potassium in your diet.

Primary Support: Potassium
***Source: Apple Cider Vinegar (Spectrum or Bragg from the health food store): 1tsp-2 Tbsp in water BID or TID (blend with a little honey to sweeten).
**Source: K-Zyme (BRC): 1-2 tablets TID
*Source: Generic Potassium

Secondary Support: Parathyroid Extract and/or Vitamin D
Use as noted previously.

Lump in Throat

Usually this is due to a potassium deficiency. Most often you're not eating enough vegetables and fruits. Check <u>Using Home Tests: Body pH</u>.

Sometimes a sense of having a lump in your throat will be due to a gall bladder or bile duct problem. Check <u>Liver/Gall Bladder</u> and <u>Using Lab Tests: Liver and Gall Bladder</u>.

Primary Support:	Potassium
***Source:	Apple Cider Vinegar (Spectrum or Bragg from the health food store) 1 tsp-2 Tbsp in water BID or TID (blend with a little honey to sweeten)
**Source:	K-Zyme (BRC): 1-2 tablets BID or TID
*Source:	Generic potassium supplement
Secondary Support:	Bile-Thinning Agent
***Source:	Beta TCP (BRC): 2 tablets after each meal
**Source:	Generic/BRC Lecithin capsules/perles: 3 BID

Dryness of Eyes, Mouth and/or Nose

This is usually a potassium deficiency, though you may need to support yourself with minerals in general. Drink more water.

Primary Support:	Potassium
***Source:	K-Zyme (BRC): 1-2 tablets BID or TID
**Source:	Generic potassium
Secondary Support:	Trace Minerals
***Source:	Celtic Salt
**Source:	Multi-Mins (BRC): 2-3 tablets a day

Phosphorus Deficiency

Joint Stiffness Upon Arising

This kind of stiffness also shows up when you haven't been moving for awhile, as in sitting in the car or working at a desk, etc. What you experience is a horrible stiffness and discomfort that clears up once you start moving around. This kind of stiffness is usually a phosphorus deficiency.

Primary Support:	Phosphorus
*** Source:	Super Phosphozyme Liquid (BRC): 1D BID/TID (decrease the dosage as stiffness clears up)
Secondary Support:	Lecithin
*** Source:	Generic/BRC Lecithin: 2-3 gelatin perles BID
Note:	Biotics lecithin is labeled Phosphatidylcholine. It is generally best to use the Liquid Phosphozyme initially, and as the stiffness clears up transition to lecithin for long-term support.

This kind of stiffness is often present in people who, because of their genetic makeup, tend to develop arteriosclerosis (clogged arteries). Using lecithin over the long haul controls this tendency and may actually even reverse arteriosclerosis. An off-white ring around the outer portion of your iris (arcus senilis) is a sure sign of arteriosclerosis. See <u>Using Lab Tests: Calcium and Phosphorus</u>.

Frequent Vomiting
This can be a sign of phosphorus deficiency. Solve the problem using the same sources of phosphorus as covered in the previous section. Also check <u>Digestion Problems</u> and <u>Liver/ Gall Bladder</u>. If chronic or severe, consult a physician.

Iron Deficiency

Tendency to Anemia
This is usually a deficiency of iron or Vitamin B12. If the whites of your eyes have a slightly blue tinge, iron deficiency is the most likely problem. Other common symptoms of iron deficiency anemia are low blood pressure, pallor of skin, cracks in nails, and restlessness or agitation. Always suspect iron-deficiency anemia with heavy menstrual periods. If you take iron and don't feel more energy after a couple of weeks, see the <u>Digestion Problems</u> and <u>Using Lab tests: Protein</u>.

Be careful with anemia, because it can mean that you are losing blood somewhere. If your anemia is severe or doesn't respond to nutritional support, consult a physician directly. <u>See Using Lab Tests: Blood Count</u>.

Primary Support:	Iron Deficiency
*** Source:	Iron-Plus (BRC): 1-2 tsp a day before meals
** Source:	Fe-Zyme (BRC): 1 tablet BID with meals
Secondary Support:	Vitamin B12 Deficiency
*** Source:	B12 2000 lozenge: 1TID between meals

Note: Iron-Plus is a very efficient and digestable form of iron. It is available from DSD International or The Elements of Health.

Whites of Eyes (Sclera) Blue
Blue sclerae are a sure sign of iron-deficiency anemia. Use the iron as in the last section.

Zinc Deficiency

White Spots on Fingernails
White spots on your fingernails usually indicate a zinc deficiency, and this is one of the most reliable ways of recognizing a need for zinc.

Primary Support:	Zinc
***Source:	Zn-Zyme forte (BRC): 1-2 tablets BID or TID
**Source:	Generic Zinc

Note: Take zinc with a meal as it can upset an empty stomach. If you take ZN-Zyme as a zinc supplement for more than 6 weeks, add a little copper (Cu-Zyme (BRC) 1-2 tablets a day).

Cuts Heal Slowly and/or Scar Easily
A zinc need, as above.

Reduced/Lost Sense of Taste and/or Smell
Also a zinc need.

Susceptible to Colds, Fevers, and/or Infections

Often a zinc deficiency, although it could be a general weakness in your immune system.

Primary Support:	General Immune Stimulant Formula
***Source:	Bio-Immunozyme (BRC): 1-2 tablets TID
**Source:	Una de Gato (AHC): 1-2 D TID
*Source:	Generic Maitake, Astragalus, or Shitake Mushroom capsules or tinctures or a combination of them.
Secondary Support:	Zinc
***Source:	Zn-Zyme forte (BRC): 1-2 tablets BID or TID
**Source:	Generic Zinc

Vitamin A Deficiency

Strong Light Irritates Eyes

This is usually <u>Low Adrenal</u>, but Vitamin A deficiency can also make your eyes sensitive to bright light.

Primary Support:	Adrenal Formula
***Source:	ADHS (BRC): 1-2 tablets BID in the morning and early afternoon
Secondary Support:	Vitamin A
***Source:	Bio-AE-Mulsion forte (BRC): 1-2 drops BID or TID
**Source:	Generic Vitamin A

Noises In Head or Ringing In Ears

Check your blood pressure first <u>Using Home Tests: Blood Pressure</u>. If your blood pressure is good, the problem is likely a Vitamin A deficiency.

Primary Support:	Vitamin A
***Source:	Bio-AE-Mulsion forte (BRC): 1-2 d BID or TID
**Source:	Generic Vitamin A

Vitamin B6 Deficiency

Burning Sensations in Mouth

This is most often a Vitamin B6 deficiency.

Always get B vitamins in their natural form. All the so-called high-potency B vitamins are crystalline-pure and won't really solve a B-vitamin deficiency. High-potency B vitamins must be phosphorylated in your liver before your body can use them. High-potency, crystalline-pure B vitamins can also cause liver stress, while natural B vitamins strengthen your liver.

Primary Support:	Phosphorylated Vitamin B6
***Source:	B6 Phosphate (BRC): 1-2 tablets TID
**Source:	Generic phosphorylated B6
Secondary Support:	Phosphorylated B Complex
***Source:	Nutritional Yeast (KAL): 2 Tbsp a day
**Source:	Bio-B-100 (BRC): 2 tablets TID with meals
*Source:	Generic phosphorylated B Complex

Numbness in Hands And Feet
This symptom is also a Vitamin B6 Deficiency. Use the same regimen as above. If this doesn't clear up, see a physician. A chiropractic physician is most likely your best choice.

Intolerant to MSG
If you get headaches, fatigue, anxiety, or other symptoms after eating food with MSG (commonly found in Chinese food), you need Vitamin B6. Support Vitamin B6 as outlined previously.

Cannot Recall Dreams
This too is a Vitamin B6 Deficiency. In fact, you can use how well you remember your dreams as a way of measuring how much B6 to take. As you begin to remember your dreams, you'll know you're taking enough (and the right kind of) B6. If your dreams become too vivid and you feel your sleep isn't sound, back off on the B6 a bit.

Many of the people I've worked with over the years remember their dreams for the first time in their lives after taking B6! They definitely get excited about this. Some people who have always dreamt in black and white begin to dream in color.

Bioflavinoid Deficiency

Frequent Nosebleeds
This is caused by dryness of the mucous membranes inside your nose or may be a bioflavinoid (synergist of Vitamin C) deficiency. To be safe, drink more water. (See The Elements of Health: Water.) Get more natural fats and oils in your diet, and avoid hydrogenated oils.

If you bruise easily, a deficiency of Vitamin K is likely. Eat more chlorophyll-rich foods (vegetables), check Liver/Gall Bladder, and supplement Vitamin K.

Primary Support:	Essential Fatty Acids (EFAs)
***Source:	Mixed EFAs (BRC): 1 Tbsp a day after a meal
**Source:	Flax oil capsules or perles (Spectrum or BRC): 3 BID after meals
*Source:	Generic Flax oil
Secondary Support:	Vitamin C with Bioflavinoids
***Source:	Bio-C Plus 1000 (BRC): 1 tablet BID
**Source:	Generic vitamin C plus bioflavinoids
Tertiary Support:	Vitamin K
*** Source:	Bio-K Mulsion (BRC): 1 drop a day
** Source:	Alfalfa (generic): 2-6 tabs BID
Note:	Keep Mixed EFAs or flax oil in the refrigerator. Don't buy a large bottle of oil; it will turn rancid before you finish it. Rancid oils have a very sharp, bitter taste and should be discarded.

Bruise Easily

Bruising usually indicates a need for bioflavinoids, but can be a problem with <u>Liver/Gall Bladder</u>. If the problem is severe, check <u>Using Lab Tests: Blood Count</u>.

Primary Support:	Vitamin C with Bioflavinoids
***Source:	Bio-C Plus 1000 (BRC): 1 tablet BID
**Source:	Generic vitamin C plus bioflavinoids
Secondary Support:	Vitamin K
*** Source:	Bio-K Mulsion (BRC): 1 drop a day
** Source:	Chlorocaps (BRC): 1-3 capsules BID
* Source:	Alfalfa (generic): 2-6 tabs BID

Vitamin E Deficiency

Muscle Cramping; Worse with Exercise

Dehydration is the most common cause of muscle cramping. Be sure you're drinking enough water and getting some natural sea salt in your diet.

If dehydration isn't the problem, look for a Vitamin E deficiency. It's best to get your Vitamin E from wheat germ oil, rather than from regular Vitamin E. If you use Vitamin E, make sure it contains mixed tocopherols.

Primary Support:	Vitamin E
***Source:	Wheat germ oil (generic; preferably made by Viobin or Spectrum) 1-3 capsules/perles: BID or 1-2 Tbsp
**Source:	E-Mulsion 200 (BRC): 1-2 capsules BID
*Source:	Generic vitamin E at 200-400 IU a day
Note:	Be careful of using high doses (above 400 IU) of Vitamin E if you are taking an anticoagulant (i.e., Coumadin) or have osteoporosis. Consult with a physician if you're considering taking more than 400 IU a day.

Heart Function

If you score 50% or less on the <u>Health Graph</u> for Heart Function, use the nutrition recommended for Heart Function for four to six weeks. If you see improvement during that time, heart function is being restored by the nutrition.

If you score high (above 50%), consult a physician and get a workup.

Better yet, consult with a functional medicine doctor who can diagnose and treat you using a functional medicine model. An Acoustic Cardiograph (ACG) usually gives more information than an EKG on how to improve heart function. The International Foundation for Nutrition and Health (IFNH) can help you find a doctor using the ACG. Call the IFNH at 858-488-8932 or visit their website at <u>www.ifnh.org</u>.

Primary Support:	Vitamin, Mineral and Enzyme Heart Support Formula
***Source:	Bio-Cardiozyme (BRC) 2 tablets TID
Secondary Support:	Phosphorylated B complex
***Source:	Bio-B 100 6 tablets TID for 1 bottle; chew
	6 tablets BID for 1 bottle; chew
	3 tablets BID thereafter; chew
Tertiary Support:	Policosanol, niacin and CoQ10 Formula
*** Source:	PCOH-Plus (BRC): 1 tab BID
Note:	Policosanol has been proven to lower cholesterol, raise HDL, and decrease platelet aggregation (reducing the risk of stroke and heart attack) without the toxicity associated with cholesterol-lowering medications.

Female Hormonal

With any female problem, always check Liver/Gall Bladder, Large Intestine, Low Thyroid, and Low Adrenal.

Use the Foundation Diet and generally avoid caffeine (especially coffee). Caffeine has been strongly connected with fibrocystic breast disease, and my personal experience in practice has been that it is also associated with premenstrual syndrome and heavy and/ or prolonged periods (dysmenorrhea).

Essential Fatty Acid Deficiency is a common underlying cause of female hormonal imbalances. Avoid hydrogenated and partially hydrogenated oils whenever possible. Read labels on packaged foods. Most will have hydrogenated oils, and with some savvy shopping you will be able to find alternatives that have natural fats and oils instead, though you may need to go to a health food store for some items. Get a lot of natural fats and oils and a couple of tablespoons of flax oil a day. (See Fatty Acids Deficiency.)

Excessive estrogen in relation to other hormones, especially progesterone, is an extremely common cause of female hormonal problems. A diet that is too high in pasta, bread, crackers, pastries, etc. promotes excessive estrogen levels. Wheat and corn are the worst culprits here. If you want grains in your diet and you're experiencing female hormonal problems, I recommend focusing on eating whole rye and oats. (See The Elements of Health: Foundation Diet.)

Estrogen is produced in body fat, so being overweight is a common reason for excessively high estrogen levels, and decreasing your body fat decreases estrogen levels. Insulin resistance causes overstimulation of female hormones and leads to the obesity that predisposes one to high estrogen levels. Suspect insulin resistance when you score high for Blood Sugar Problems, and confirm insulin resistance by referring to Using Lab Tests: Blood Fats.

Pesticides and plastics contain compounds that act like estrogen (xenobiotics), and commercial (non-organic) animal products such as meat, chicken, milk, and eggs have estrogen residues in them. Buy organically produced animal products and produce whenever you can. Avoid foods and drinks that have been packaged or stored in plastic containers and be particularly careful of cooking foods in plastic containers (boiling or microwave).

Phytoestrogens from soy actually decrease overall estrogen activity when estrogen levels are too high, and block the adverse effect of xenobiotics (estrogen-mimicking compounds from plastics and pesticides). Soy has been controversial because of excess estrogen being a factor in estrogen-dependent cancers. This comes from a misunderstanding of the strength of soy's estrogen activity, which is much lower than the estrogen your body produces. Soy can be used to decrease overall estrogen activity when it is too high by binding the receptor sites for estrogen. This prevents the estrogen your body produces from acting as fully, and decreases the effect xenobiotics have on your estrogen activity. When estrogen levels are too low, soy's mild estrogen activity can control hot flashes.

Primary Support:	Female Balancing Formula
***Source:	Equifem (BRC): 1-2 tablets BID or TID
**Source:	Lunazon (AHC): 1-2D BID/TID or 1-2 caps BID/TID
Note:	Consider using both Equifem and Lunazon together for stronger support and balancing of female hormones. PMT (BRC) is the vegetarian form of Equifem; same dosage.
Secondary Support:	Soy Phyto-Estrogens
***Source:	Soy Isoflavones (BRC): 1-2 capsules BID or TID
**Source:	Gamoctapro (BRC): 2 heaping Tbsp once or twice a day
*Source:	Generic Soy Protein Powder or 8 oz of soy milk a day (I recommend Edensoy® Vanilla)

Female problems can be very complex. If you don't see improvement on follow-up Health Graphs, get the Expanded Female Hormonal Panel done. Read Using Lab Tests: Specialty Tests To Consider to help solve the problem, or consult a physician directly.

Male Hormonal

Prostate Problems
If your score is high here and you haven't had your prostate checked, now is the time. Get a digital exam and a PSA test. When the Creatinine from your lab work is 1.2 or higher, it correlates very strongly with prostate disease. To have a healthy prostate, eat from the Foundation Diet, get more exercise, and have sex more often.

Fatty Acids Deficiency and Large Intestine Problems complicate prostate problems. Support these areas as needed. Use Kegel exercises as covered in Low Libido/Impotence to improve circulation to the prostate.

Primary Support: Prostate Formula
***Source: Palmetto Plus (BRC): 1-2 capsules BID
**Source: Generic Prostate Formula including Saw Palmetto

Secondary Support: Pumpkin Seed Oil
***Source: Pumpkin Seed Oil (generic): 1-2 Tbsp a day

Tertiary Support: Soy Phyto-estrogens (See Female Hormonal)
***Source: Soy Isoflavones (BRC): 1-2 capsules BID or TID
**Source: Gamoctapro (BRC): 2 heaping Tbsp once or twice a day
*Source: Generic Soy Protein Powder

Low Libido (Men and Women)/ Impotence

Prostate problems are a common cause of low libido/impotence. Other common causes of low libido/impotence are High Autonomic, Low Adrenal, Low Pituitary, Blood Sugar Problems, Liver/Gall Bladder, and Large Intestine. Support these areas as indicated. Also, check your blood pressure and screen for diabetes with a glycated hemoglobin test. (See Using Lab Tests: Energy.) Detoxification programs and fasting can make a remarkable difference. (See The Elements of Health: Detoxification and Fasting.)

Kegel exercises are very useful to increase sexual sensitivity and intensity of orgasm for men and women. Kegels are also helpful for incontinence and to make for stronger erections. To do the Kegel exercise, tighten the muscles that you use when you want to hold back your urine. Squeeze these muscles tightly and hold for a moment before releasing. When done properly, you can feel a slight forward movement of the lower tip of your sacrum (lower aspect of your pelvis in the middle). Work up to 100 repetitions twice a day or more. These exercises can be done anytime, while sitting, driving, standing, etc. Be consistent; it may take a few weeks of consistent exercise before you see changes.

Primary Support: High Autonomic Herbal Formula
*** Source: Parasympa (DR): 1-2D BID/TID in water

Secondary Support: Sexual Tonic Herbs
*** Source: Sumacazon (AHC): 2D BID/TID
** Source: B-Vital (BRC): 1-2 capsules BID

Note: Using Sumacazon (AHC), B-Vital (BRC), and Warrior (AHC) together can be very useful. For the Warrior, use the same dosage as for Sumacazon.

Tertiary Support: Male Glandular
*** Source: Cytozyme M (BRC): 2 tabs BID/TID; chew

Note: Though Cytozyme M was formulated for men, it is appropriate and useful for women with high estrogen and/or low libido.

General Principles

Home Tests

- Pulse
- Blood Pressure
- Body Temperature
- Body pH
- Zinc Taste Test (ZTT)
- Oxidation Stress Test
- Calcium (Sulkowitch) Test
- Sodium (Koenisburg) Test

Home tests allow you to measure the status of your health, direct your selfcare based on information gained through testing, and objectively evaluate the results of any therapy you use based on the results you get when retesting. You control your own health; only you know whether a therapy does or doesn't work for you.

At the end of this section is a sample of the form used to record the results of successive tests for comparing your results. Use it as an example. The same form can be found in the back of this workbook. Use it to make copies. The Home Test Form is also included on the accompanying CD-ROM for printing from a computer.

Pulse

Taking your pulse costs you nothing, is easy to do, and gives you an ongoing measure of your health.

Count your pulse for a full minute to get a good reading. Ideally, it should be between 60 and 80 beats a minute, except for well-trained athletes who tend to have a pulse lower than 60 beats a minute because the stroke volume of their heart is greater than most people. Greater stroke volume means the heart doesn't need to beat as often to get enough oxygen-carrying blood around to meet the body's needs.

Interpreting Pulse

Pulse Greater than 80 Beats a Minute	Pulse Less than 60 Beats a Minute
• Sympathetic Dominance	• Parasympathetic Dominant
• Vitamin G Deficiency	• B Vitamin Deficiency
• Calcium/Phosphorus Imbalance (<2.4)	• Calcium/Phosphorus Imbalance (>2.4)
• Cholesterol and/or Triglycerides too high	• Normal for well-trained athletes
• High Adrenal	• Low Adrenal
• High Pituitary	• Low Pituitary
• High Thyroid	• Low Thyroid
• Food/Environmental Allergies/Sensitivities	• Food/Environmental Allergies/Sensitivities

Interpreting Fast Pulse

Greater than 80 Beats a Minute	What to Do
Sympathetic Dominant	Check your score for <u>High Autonomic</u> from the <u>Health Graph</u>.
Vitamin G Deficiency	Check your score for <u>Vitamin G Deficiency</u> from the <u>Health Graph</u>.
Calcium/Phosphorus Imbalance (<2.4)	Check your <u>Calcium/Phosphorus</u> balance (<u>Using Lab Tests: Calcium and Phosphorus</u>).
Cholesterol and/or Triglycerides too high	Check <u>Using Lab Tests: Blood Fats</u>.
High Adrenal	Check your score in that section of the <u>Health Graph</u> and <u>Stress and Life</u>.
High Pituitary	See that section of the <u>Health Graph</u> and support, if indicated.
High Thyroid	See that section of the <u>Health Graph</u> and support, if indicated.
Food/Environmental Allergies/ Sensitivities	• See <u>Allergies</u> section of the <u>Health Graph</u> and support, if indicated. • Avoid milk, milk products, all bread, pasta, anything with grains, eggs, soy products, nightshades (tomatoes, potatoes, yams, sweet potatoes, eggplant and peppers), and citrus for 1-2 weeks to see if you feel better and your pulse normalizes. If so, add one food back in at a time every 2 days and keep a record of how you feel. If you feel worse and/or your pulse goes back up, you're allergic to that food. • Consider getting tested for allergies as indicated in <u>Using Lab Tests: Specialty Tests to Consider</u>.

Interpreting Slow Pulse

Pulse Less than 60 Beats a Minute	What to Do
Parasympathetic Dominant	Check your score for <u>Low Autonomic</u> from the <u>Health Graph</u>.
B Vitamin Deficiency	Check your score for <u>B Vitamin Deficiency</u> from the <u>Health Graph</u>.
Calcium/Phosphorus Imbalance (>2.4)	Check the <u>Calcium and Phosphorus</u> in <u>Using Lab Tests Low Pituitary</u> of the <u>Health Graph</u>, if indicated.
Low Thyroid	Refer to <u>Low Thyroid</u> from the <u>Health Graph</u>.
Low Adrenal	Refer to <u>Low Adrenal</u> from the <u>Health Graph</u>.
Food-Environmental Allergies/Sensitivities	Graph and support, if indicated. • See the <u>Allergies</u> section of the <u>Health Graph</u>. • Avoid milk and milk products, all bread and pasta and anything else with grains in them. Eggs, soy products, nightshades (tomatoes, potatoes, yams and sweet potatoes, eggplant, and peppers), and citrus for 1-2 weeks to see if you feel better and your pulse goes up. If so, add one food back in at a time every 2 days and keep a record of how you feel; if you feel worse, you're allergic to that food. • Consider getting tested for allergies, as indicated in <u>Using Lab Tests: Specialty Tests to Consider</u>.

Blood Pressure

I recommend an automatic, digital blood pressure cuff (sphygmomanometer) costing between $80-$100. The cheapest models usually don't give precise readings, and the top-end models have bells and whistles you really don't need. The blood pressure unit you buy should include a book which provides a basic understanding of blood pressure and instructions on taking readings.

Taking your blood pressure gives two numbers. **The upper number is called the systolic**, and **the lower number is called the diastolic.** To get the most out of what your blood pressure can tell you, take it in three different positions: sitting, lying down, and standing. First, take your blood pressure sitting; then lie down for 3 minutes and take your blood pressure again; then stand and immediately retake your blood pressure.

Here's what you should find:

Blood Pressure Dynamics		
Position	**Ideal Findings**	**Meaning**
Sitting	120/80	Good circulation, oxygen, and nutrients are getting to the tissues of your body.
Lying	Diastolic decreases	Proper kidney (secondarily liver) function.
Standing	Systolic increases	Good function of adrenal glands.

Interpreting Blood Pressure

Position	Result	What to Do	(P) = See Pulse section
Sitting	Above 86 Diastolic	<ul><li>See Liver/Gall Bladder from the Health Graph.</li><li>Make sure you're well-hydrated.</li><li>Avoid commercial salt.</li><li>Cholesterol and/or triglycerides too high (P).</li><li>Need for exercise (consider a trainer).</li><li>High Autonomic</li><li>Vitamin G Deficiency</li><li>High Adrenal</li><li>High Pituitary</li><li>High Thyroid</li><li>Food/Environmental Allergies</li></ul>	
	Below 76 Diastolic	<ul><li>High Autonomic</li><li>Vitamin B Deficiency</li><li>Deficiency of natural salts (Celtic Salt).</li><li>Dehydration</li><li>Low Adrenal</li><li>Low Thyroid</li><li>Low Pituitary</li><li>Food/Environmental Allergies (P)</li></ul>	
	Above 130 Systolic	<ul><li>Same as Above 86 Diastolic.</li></ul>	
	Below 114 Systolic	<ul><li>Same as Below 76 Diastolic.</li></ul>	
Lying	Diastolic increases or stays the same	<ul><li>Kidney function impaired; see Using Lab Tests: Electrolytes.</li><li>Liver function impaired; See Liver/Gall Bladder. from Health Graph and Using Lab Tests: Liver and Gall Bladder.</li><li>Dehydration</li></ul>	
	Diastolic decreases	<ul><li>Proper kidney (secondarily liver) function.</li></ul>	
Standing	Systolic increases 4-10 mmHg	<ul><li>Normal; good adrenal function.</li></ul>	
	Systolic increases more than 4-10 mmHg	<ul><li>High Autonomic</li><li>Vitamin G Deficiency</li><li>High Adrenal</li><li>High Pituitary</li><li>High Thyroid</li><li>Food-Environmental Allergies (P)</li></ul>	
	Systolic stays the same or decreases	<ul><li>Low Adrenal</li><li>B Vitamin Deficiency</li><li>Low Pituitary</li></ul>	

Body Temperature

Temperature mostly tells you about your metabolism. A low temperature indicates your metabolism is too low. A high temperature indicates your metabolism is too high.

Digital thermometers don't work well. I've bought the professional models to use in my office and I can't depend on them, and the inexpensive ones you get at the drug store definitely don't work. Though getting hard to find, you need to use a mercury thermometer to get accurate temperature readings. Call *The Elements of Health*, 866-563-4256, if you can't find a mercury thermometer locally.

Chart your temperature for four days. Shake your thermometer down before going to bed. When you wake up in the morning before rising, put the thermometer under your arm and leave it there for 10 minutes. Chart your temperature for 4 days and then average the results.

Interpreting Temperature	
Temperature	**What to Do**
97.8–98.2	● Balanced metabolism
Above 98.4	● Acute infection. See physician if temperature is above 102, if the fever is over 3 days, or if you become dehydrated despite using lots of fluids. See Using Lab Tests: Blood Count. ● Chronic infections (Usually these infections are viral). See Using Lab Tests: Blood Count. ● High Thyroid ● High Autonomic ● Vitamin G Deficiency ● High Adrenal
Below 97.8	● Low Thyroid ● Low Adrenal ● Vitamin B Deficiency

Body pH

Balancing your body pH is like magic for the way your body works! Adjusting your diet will usually balance pH and help normalize your body chemistry (hormone, immune, and enzyme systems).

Do all those shelves of diet books just make you more confused about diet? They all claim they have the answer for you. Yet some say you should eat meat, cheese, and eggs; some promote vegetarianism or even a veganism (no animal products); some say you need almost all raw fruits and veggies; some say grains are the answer; some say you should eat according to your blood type.

Many authors claim their diet is the be-all, end-all, and cure-all. But no single diet works for everyone. The trick is to figure out which is right for you.

First, check your body pH, the acid-alkaline balance which controls every chemical reaction in your body. Balancing this one aspect of your body chemistry will make a huge difference in how your body works.

Check both urine and saliva pH first thing in the morning using pH paper strips (Hydrion pH 4-9), which you can buy from chemistry supply stores or *The Elements of Health*, 866-563-4256.

Catch some of your first morning urine in a paper cup and dip in a strip of the pH paper. Compare the color of the pH paper to the reference chart included with the paper, and chart the result.

Check your saliva pH by putting a strip on your tongue and holding the strip against the roof of your mouth with your tongue for half a minute. Check the color of the pH strip against the reference colors and chart the result.

Do this for four mornings, then average the findings for saliva and urine pH before interpreting the result.

Ideal Body pH (Acid-Alkaline Balance)
Saliva pH = 7.2
Urine pH = 6.4

Interpreting Body pH

Saliva Finding	Urine Finding	What to Do
pH < 7.2	pH < 6.4	Increase fruits and vegetables
pH > 7.2	pH > 6.4	Increase meats and eggs
pH < 7.2	pH > 6.4	Increase fats and oils
pH > 7.2	pH < 6.4	Increase grains

> greater than < less than

Be patient. Balancing your pH may take months, but stick with the changes indicated from the pH testing. Your pH indicates the ideal diet for you, based on your unique body chemistry. Follow it and the pH will balance, and you'll feel better as your body functions better.

Balancing Acid pH

Changing a pH that is acidic for both saliva and urine can be difficult. You may be working to reverse the results of eating too little fruits and vegetables in your diet for many, many years. And it can take an incredible amount of vegetables to make the needed change in your body chemistry and pH. A hint: when you think you're eating more vegetables than you could possibly need, you're getting close to enough.

Getting a juicer and using 8 to 16 ounces of fresh vegetable juices once or twice a day can really speed up the results. My favorite is carrot, celery, and beet juice. Fresh wheatgrass juice is also a great approach to straightening out your acid-alkaline balance.

Another approach that works well is to use apple cider vinegar. Make sure you go to the health food store to get the apple cider vinegar. My favorite brands are Bragg's or Spectrum.

Put one or two tablespoons of apple cider vinegar in a glass of water. This makes a tart, refreshing drink that does a great job raising your saliva and urine pH. You can put a little honey in with the apple cider vinegar to sweeten it a bit. I use a jar with a lid, so I can shake it and get the honey to mix in easily.

The Zinc Taste Test

I test virtually everyone who comes in to my office for Zinc Deficiency and find that the majority are deficient.

Without enough zinc, you can't make the enzymes needed to digest the food you eat, you can't make neurotransmitters like serotonin, dopamine, and gamma-amino butyric acid (GABA), your liver can't make the enzymes it needs to function, you can't make hormones (including male and female hormones), and the cells of your body can't divide efficiently so your body can repair and regenerate itself.

Common signs of Zinc Deficiency are poor immune function, loss of sense of taste or smell, wounds that heal slowly, acne, reduced sex drive, prostate hypertrophy, female and male hormone problems, depression, agitation, and anxiety, chronic yeast infections, macular degeneration, hair loss, dandruff, premature graying of the hair, and white spots on the fingernails.

This deficiency is common. Foods grown commercially are usually lacking zinc due to depletion of soils caused by failure to till under soils, rotate crops, or use natural fertilizers. Zinc is further lost when foods are processed or refined.

Many people need far more zinc than the recommended daily allowance (RDA) of 15 mg, with a great number of my patients finding their health improves when using as much as 150 mg a day on a regular basis. A need for lots of zinc seems to be genetically determined or, said another way, to run in the family. My experience has been that if the daughter I'm working with has chronic depression due to low serotonin levels resulting from a zinc need, the mom's depression will likely be alleviated with zinc, too.

Luckily, zinc is one of the few nutrients you can test for without needing an expensive blood test. The Zinc Taste Test is simple, quick, inexpensive, and accurate. You can order the solution (Aqueous Zinc) for doing the test from *The Elements of Health*, or DSD International at 800-232-3183, or 602-944-0104.

To do the test, hold two teaspoons of the solution in your mouth for thirty seconds. The taste of the solution will be very strong if your body has sufficient zinc levels. If you're deficient in zinc, you will either taste nothing, or the taste will be very faint.

Interpreting the Zinc Taste Test (ZTT)

Finding	Grade	Meaning	What to Do
No taste or tastes like water.	1	Marked zinc deficiency	Iron/copper-free multiple vitamin/mineral supplement **and** additional zinc (for 150 mg total) until ZTT of 4.
No immediate taste though a vague taste develops over time.	2	Moderate zinc deficiency	Iron/copper-free multiple-vitamin/ mineral supplement **and** additional zinc (for 75 mg total) until ZTT of 4.
Slight initial taste that becomes stronger over time; may be unpleasant.	3	Mild zinc deficiency	Iron/copper-free multiple vitamin/ mineral supplement to increase absorption of zinc.
Very strong, unpleasant and immediate taste.	4	Zinc sufficient	No supplementation needed, or use balanced multiple-vitamin/mineral supplement.

Note: Don't take large doses of zinc over a long period of time without balancing it with some iron and copper. If you're using high doses (above 50 mg) of zinc for more than two months, take a multiple vitamin that includes iron and copper.

Deficiencies of iron and copper are usually due to poor absorption, not because of inadequate intake. The results of too little zinc and too much iron and copper are nervousness, anxiety, inability to concentrate, fatigue, heart disease, and menstrual imbalances in women.

Taking a multiple-vitamin and -mineral formula without iron and copper helps optimize the absorption of zinc that is present and restores the balance between iron, copper, and zinc. A very effective iron/copper-free multiple-vitamin/mineral supplement is Iron and Copper Free Bio-Multiplus (BRC).

The zinc supplement I prefer is ZN-Zyme Forte (BRC). ZN-Zyme Forte has 25 mg of zinc per tablet.

The Oxidation Stress Test

Every cell of your body produces free-radical compounds as a normal part of cellular metabolism. It's like the exhaust from your car; you can't produce energy in the engine to make your car run without also producing the exhaust. They go together. So too, every cell of your body produces exhaust as free radicals.

Free radicals, if unchecked, destroy the cell wall and the structures within the cell. As cells become more and more damaged from the effects of free radicals, they function abnormally, and they age.

The higher the levels of free radicals are in your body, the faster the damage takes place. Oxidation is the state of your body's free-radical levels. High oxidation levels (high free-radical levels) cause more tissue damage than low oxidation levels (low free-radical levels).

Most of the effects we associate with aging can be attributed to cell damage caused by free radicals. One of the most consistent factors found in older centenarians is their relatively low level of free radicals. Many researchers and physicians have proposed that free-radical damage is the primary cause of aging, and that controlling free-radical levels is the single most important strategy for being more vital and healthy as you age.

Inflammatory conditions such as allergies, arthritis, colitis, irritable bowel syndrome, sinusitis, bursitis, myositis, etc. are caused, at least in part, by free radicals. Excessive free-radical levels in your body may complicate injuries that heal slowly or remain inflamed.

Antioxidants are compounds in your body that control free-radical levels by breaking them down into harmless compounds. A number of enzymes are involved in this process. The more important ones are superoxide dismutase, glutathione peroxidase, methionine reductase, and catalase. Don't worry, you don't have to remember them; there's no test.

The vitamins and minerals known as antioxidants play a role in producing, protecting, or aiding the antioxidant enzymes. The primary antioxidant nutrients are Vitamins A, C, E, and F (essential fatty acids) and the minerals copper, selenium, sulfur, and zinc.

Optimizing antioxidant levels is one of the most important things you do to protect your health. There are lab tests to determine what your antioxidant levels are, but they're rather exotic and expensive.

A much simpler and less expensive way to measure your antioxidant levels is the Oxidation Stress Test. This test measures the level of oxidation present in your body tissues from a urine sample. A small amount of urine is placed in a glass ampoule containing a reagent, and if high levels of by-products are present in your urine from oxidation of your body tissues, the solution will turn red. With lower levels of oxidation, the solution will turn various shades of pink.

Using the Oxidation Stress Test allows you to simply and inexpensively test your body's oxidation levels and antioxidant need. Redoing the test periodically allows you to make sure that tissue oxidation is being controlled, an essential component of selfcare. The test will also help you find the antioxidant formula or blend of antioxidants your body needs to control oxidation.

You may need to experiment a bit until you find the best combination for you. This way, you are able to determine your unique makeup and the approach that best controls your body's oxidation. As long as you continue to use a combination that controls oxidation for you (which may change a little depending on diet, environment, stress, etc.), you'll do great.

Doing the Oxidation Stress Test

Reagent-filled glass ampoules for the Oxidation Stress Test are available from *The Elements of Health*, 866-563-4256. Included with the ampoule is a chart for evaluating the results of the test and a plastic bulb with an attached tube called a pipette. The pipette allows you to precisely measure your urine (1ml) before combining with the reagent.

Don't take any supplements the day before doing this test. Many supplements can color your urine and interfere with interpretation of the test. This is particularly true of the B vitamins, especially B2 (riboflavin), and Vitamin C. Also, some medications may alter the color of your urine and affect your ability to interpret the Oxidation Stress Test accurately.

Do this test from urine passed when you first urinate after arising in the morning (first morning urine). Retain enough of that urine directly into a disposable cup (not from urine in the toilet bowl) to fill half of the cup. Break off the top of the glass ampoule (it's not as hard to do as it might look) and place one milliliter (1ml) of urine into the ampoule using the plastic pipette. There is a one-milliliter mark on the pipette. Let the ampoule sit for five minutes and then hold it up to the interpretation card to evaluate the result. Match the color of the solution in the ampoule to the appropriate color on the card and chart the result. Don't let the solution sit for more than five minutes, or the test result won't be accurate.

The results will vary from no change to bright red. The less change there is in the color of your urine, the less oxidation is taking place in the cells of your body. If the color of your urine doesn't change, you don't need to supplement antioxidants. With the progression of color change, you will increase the level of antioxidant support. As you retest over time, you can adjust the amount of antioxidant support appropriate to your need.

Warning: The reagent used in this test is toxic. Do not ingest or inhale it. Do not add the contents of the vial to the test urine. Keep out of the reach of children. In case of accidental ingestion, or if the contents of the vial get into your eyes, call a physician immediately.

Interpreting the Oxidation Stress Test

Finding	Meaning	What to Do
+3 Marked Oxidation	Marked Antioxidant Deficiency	• Bio-Cyanidins (BRC): 1-2 tabs BID • GSH Plus (BRC): 1 cap TID • Mixed Ascorbate Powder (BRC): 3,000–8,000 mg (3-8 grams) or to bowel tolerance (take increasing dosage until loose stools occur and then decrease dosage slightly). • Bioprotect (BRC): 1-3 BID
+2 Moderate Oxidation	Definite Antioxidant Deficiency	• Mixed Ascorbate Powder (BRC): 2,000-4,000 mg (2-4 grams) or to bowel tolerance (take increasing dosage until loose stools occur and then decrease dosage slightly). • Bioprotect (BRC): 1-3 BID
+1 Low Oxidation	Probable Antioxidant Deficiency	• Vitamin C with bioflavinoids (generic): 1,000-2,000 mg (1-2 grams) or Bio C Plus 1000 (BRC) at 1-2 a day • Bioprotect (BRC): 1-2 BID
0 No Oxidation	Great!	• Celebrate!

If you don't get an adequate response with the above regimen, consider the following:
- Antioxidant need increases with exposure to environmental toxins. (See The Elements of Health: Non-Toxic Environment.)
- Antioxidant need increases with toxicity from the intestines. (See The Elements of Health: Detoxification and Fasting.)
- Vegetables and fruits are natural sources of antioxidants; make sure you're getting enough in your diet. (See Using Home Tests: Body pH.)
- It is often difficult to get enough fruits and vegetables by eating them alone; you may need to use fresh vegetable juices, also. (See The Elements of Health: Juices.)
- Make sure you get enough sulfur in your diet. Eat onions, garlic, horseradish, ginger, cayenne, and eggs.
- Essential Fatty Acid Deficiency may be a cause. (See Fatty Acids Deficiency.)
- Check the Zinc Taste Test to determine your zinc need and support accordingly.

Interpreting the Oxidation Stress Test

Problem	Solution	What to Do
Need for Specialty Antioxidants	Pycnogenols	• Bio-Cyanidins (BRC): 1-2 tabs BID • Generic Pycnogenols
	Glutathione, Acetylcysteine, and Glycine	• GSH Plus (BRC): 1 cap TID • Generic sources of these nutrients
	Plant Antioxidants	• Wheatgrass juice (generic) • Dismuzyme Granules (BRC): 1-3 tsp a day • Wheatgrass, Oat, Rye and/or Barley Grass concentrate (Use Pure Synergy Powder (TSC): 1-2 Tbsp per day)
Need for Higher Concentrations of Antioxidant Nutrients	Vitamin A	• Bio-AE Mulsion Forte (BRC): 2-4 drops TID (not to be used while pregnant) • Generic Vitamin A (25,000-50,000 IU; not to be used while pregnant)
	Vitamin C	• See preceding table for <u>Oxidation Stress Test</u>.
	Vitamin E	• E-Mulsion 200 at 200-400 IU per day • Generic Vitamin E at 200-400 IU per day
	Selenium	• SE-Zyme Forte (BRC): 1-2 TID • Aqueous Selenium (BRC): 1d TID • Generic selenium
	Zinc	• Check the <u>Zinc Taste Test</u>. • ZN Zyme Forte: 1-2 tabs BID/TID with meals • Generic zinc up to 150 mg per day

The Calcium Test

Calcium is an essential mineral and electrolyte. Calcium is the main supportive element in your bones and teeth, and accounts for about 70% of the weight of bone in your body. About 99% of the calcium in your body is bound in bone. The other 1% regulates muscle contraction (including heart muscle), allows nerve conduction, affects blood clotting, controls hormone secretion, and plays a role in enzyme function.

The primary factors regulating calcium levels are Vitamin D and parathyroid hormone. Your stomach must have a very acid pH for absorption of calcium (the calcium in antacids is not available for absorption) and the villi of your small intestine must be healthy for absorption.

The usual results of calcium deficiency are irritability and nervousness, insomnia, osteoporosis, high blood pressure, and muscle cramping. Calcium also plays an important role in blood clotting, control of allergies and immune response, and the health of your skin.

Often when calcium levels test low, the real problem is absorption of calcium in the intestines. Check the Digestive Function section from the Health Graph and support as indicated. Also, see Absorption in the Nutritional Deficiency section of the Health Graph.

Good food sources of calcium are milk and milk products (yogurt, cheese, etc.), leafy green vegetables, oats, sesame seeds, almonds, and fish (salmon, sardines).

There is a simple and inexpensive test for calcium levels. Using a urine sample, the test measures the calcium that normally spills into your urine when the levels are high enough in your bloodstream. In many ways, this is a more accurate measurement of your calcium balance than a blood test.

Do this test by mixing equal parts of urine and Sulkowitch reagent in a test tube. Calcium test reagent and test tubes are available from *The Elements of Health*, 866-563-4256. Shake the test tube gently to mix the reagent and urine together. Let the test tube sit for two minutes and then interpret according to following table.

Interpreting the Calcium Test (Sulkowitch Test)

Finding	Grade	Meaning	What to Do
No cloudiness	1	Marked calcium deficiency	1) Digestion Problems 2) Check Absorption from the Nutritional Deficiency section of the Health Graph. 3) Bio-D Mulsion (BRC): 1-2 drops BID or TID (decrease dosage as calcium levels improve). 4) Ca/Mg Plus (BRC): 1-2 tabs TID before meals.
Slight cloudiness; can easily read markings on test tube.	2	Moderate calcium deficiency	1) Ca/Mg Zyme: 2-3 tablets TID on an empty stomach. 2) Digestion Problems and Absorption from the Nutritional Deficiency section of the Health Graph.
Moderately cloudy; can barely read markings.	3	Normal calcium levels	Nothing.
Very cloudy; unable to read markings.	4	Excess calcium levels	1) Decrease or stop calcium supplements. 2) Check for kidney function from lab test; see Using Lab Tests: Electrolytes. 3) Look to refined foods in your diet; they tend to be fortified with Vitamin D and are a common cause of too much of this vitamin in the diet. 4) Ca/Mg Plus (BRC): 1-2 tabs TID before meals (parathyroid glandular in Ca/Mg Plus helps regulate calcium levels).

The Sodium Test

Salt is not bad for you. What's bad are too much or too little or not the right kind. Your adrenal glands and kidneys normally regulate the amount of salt in your body. If the kidneys and adrenal glands are functioning normally, when you have too much salt, your kidneys excrete it; when you have too little salt, your kidneys retain it.

Salt is essential for your body to function. Simply put, no salt, no life. If you haven't read about Celtic salt already, see The Elements of Health: Salt.

Aldosterone, one of the primary hormones from your adrenal glands, regulates the amount of salts excreted in your urine. Measuring the salt (sodium) in your urine is a simple, inexpensive, and useful way to understand how your adrenal glands are functioning.

Collect your urine in a paper cup. Use the dropper to place ten drops of urine in a test tube. Then place one drop of potassium chromate into the test tube and gently shake it to mix the solution. Then drop silver nitrate into the test tube drop by drop until a brick-red color develops. Count the number of drops you add. As you get close to the end, point the solution will turn red, but will return to a milky yellow color as you gently shake the test tube. Write down how many drops of silver nitrate you used to get the solution to turn and stay red. If you go to 50 drops and the solution hasn't yet turned brick red, stop the test and mark the result as "50+."

A word of caution: Be careful with silver nitrate; anything you drop it onto will be permanently stained.

The reagents for doing the sodium test are available from *The Elements of Health*, 866-563-4256.

Interpreting the Sodium Test (Koenisburg Test)	
Finding	**Meaning**
18-22 Drops	Optimal
24-50+ Drops	Low Adrenal Excessive salt consumption Kidney dysfunction (See Using Lab Tests: Electrolytes)
1-16 Drops	High Adrenal Low Adrenal (Stage II exhaustion) Salt-restricted diet Kidney dysfunction (See Using Lab Tests: Electrolytes)

Home Tests Form

Name:

Date:				
Pulse (Ideal Range: 50-70 BPM)				
Sitting Blood Pressure (Ideal: 120/80) Ideal Range: 114-130/76-86				
Lying Blood Pressure				
Lying Blood Pressure Change (+/-) Norm: Slight drop in Diastolic				
Standing Blood Pressure				
Standing Blood Pressure Change (+/-) Norm: Increase Systolic 4-10mmHg <4mmHg = Low Adrenal >10mmHg = High Adrenal, High Pituitary or Sympathetic Dominant				
Saliva pH (Norm: 7.2)				
Urine pH (Norm: 6.5)				
Temperature (4-day average) Ideal Range: 97.8-98.2 <97.8 = Low Thyroid, Low Pituitary, Low Adrenal, or Vitamin B Deficiency >98.2 = High Thyroid, High Pituitary, acute or chronic infection.				
Zinc Taste Test 1 = No taste = Marked zinc-deficiency 2 = Slight, delayed taste = Zinc-deficiency 3 = Distinct taste = Slight zinc-deficiency 4 = Very strong/unpleasant taste = Good				
Oxidation Stress Test +3 = Marked antioxidant need +2 = Definite antioxidant need +1 = Probable antioxidant need 0 = No antioxidant need				
Urine Calcium (Sulkowitch Test) 1 = Clear = Marked calcium deficiency 2 = Slightly cloudy = Calcium deficiency 3 = Moderately cloudy = Normal 4 = Milky = Excess calcium				
Urine Sodium (Koenisburg Test) 18-22 = Normal 24 or greater = Low Adrenal 16 or lower = High Adrenal or Low Adrenal at Stage II exhaustion				

General Principles

Using laboratory findings (primarily blood work) gives you an objective basis from which to build your health and wellbeing. You will learn more about your health than you ever thought possible once you begin to compare your lab findings with the tables and flowcharts in this section. Illness will no longer be a mystery; what to do to in order to restore your health will be a certainty for you.

Traditionally, interpreting lab findings was the physician's domain. Now, this workbook shows you how to read your lab work results and understand how your body functions, learn what needs to be done to restore less-than-optimal body functions, and measure the results when you retest. All you need to do is go through the process step-by-step. Before you know it, you'll be able to do this consistently and accurately, and it won't take much time or effort.

Once you own these tools, you will never have to rely on someone else's claims about any medicine, nutrition supplements, diet, or therapy. You will know without a doubt for yourself what works and what doesn't work for you.

Getting Lab Tests

You have two sources for lab work: your doctor or directly from a lab.

Ask your doctor for copies of recent lab work (preferably within the last three months) or request that your doctor order lab work for you. If the doctor resists, remember, you have a legal right to copies. You may need to sign a records release form, which is common and something I do in my practice.

Some diagnostic laboratories will permit you to have your lab work done without an order from a doctor ("direct to the consumer" lab testing). This allows you to call the shots — and that's how it should be.

I recommend a lab panel that includes the following tests: SMAC 24 (chemistry panel), GGTP, Magnesium, CBC (complete blood count), Lipid Panel, and Thyroid Panel (including T3 Uptake, T4, T7 and TSH).

On the following page is a table of these tests with discussion.

Recommended Lab Panel

Test	Discussion
SMAC 24 (Chemistry Panel)	Includes tests for kidney and liver function, minerals, proteins, and energy production.
GGTP	An important test for understanding liver and gall bladder function.
Serum Magnesium	Very important mineral and electrolyte test.
CBC (Complete Blood Count)	Tests for anemias, immune function, allergies, and infections.
Lipid Panel	Screens for heart disease risk, insulin resistance, diabetes, and carbohydrate tolerance.
Thyroid Panel (T3 Uptake, T4, T7 and TSH)	Screens for regulation of metabolism.

Charting Lab Tests

Begin by requesting copies of your lab work from your doctor or directly from the lab. Chart the results in the Lab Findings Form from Appendices: Forms, and highlight values that are higher or lower than normal. Preferably use two different-colored highlighting pens, one for the high and one for the low values.

It is not the purpose of this workbook to diagnose or treat pathological illnesses. If any of your lab values on the Lab Findings Form meet or exceed the listed alarm value for any lab test result, see a physician for further exams and recommendations!

Study your charted lab findings to get a feel of the overall picture of how your body functions and what needs work. Then return to the findings for specific information and actions to take.

Follow the directions and suggestions related to your lab findings. Repeat lab tests in 6 to 12 weeks to get new values. Improvements in your lab results will verify the improvement in your body functions. That's what functional medicine is all about — restoring health by restoring body function.

If follow-up lab results indicate your health is not improving (especially if you've done several follow-up labs without results), the needed work may be outside the scope of this workbook. Most of the time you will see and feel fantastic changes.

Complete another <u>Health Graph</u>, re-check your home tests, and re-evaluate your new lab work. From there you'll have an idea what has changed and what hasn't. Use the same criteria as the first time around; focus on the main points from the <u>Health Graph</u> and the <u>Home Tests</u>. Take that information and go over your lab report. Pick one to three things to work on.

Re-check your lab again in 6–12 weeks. If you're not seeing the kind of changes you expect on the follow-up lab reports, consult a physician.

Refer to <u>Using The Workbook: Glossary</u> for interpretation keys to the recommendations and tables that follow.

For clarity and convenience, you may want to print <u>Using The Workbook: Glossary</u> to use while working through this section of the workbook. This chart appears on page 33 of this workbook and is also on the CD-ROM included with the printed version.

Lab Findings Form (Page 1 of 2)

Lab Tests

Name: _____ **Lab Sheet #:** _____

Date:				
Electrolyte Balance				
Magnesium	>2.0			
Potassium	4.0–4.5			
Sodium	135–142			
Chloride	100–106			
Energy				
Glucose	80–95			
Glycated Hemoglobin	<7			
Carbon Dioxide	26-31			
Protein				
BUN	10–16			
Creatinine	.8-1.1			
Uric Acid	(F) 3.0–5.5 (M) 3.5–5.9			
Total Protei n	6.8–7.4			
Albumin	4.0–4.9			
Globulin	2.4–2.8			
Blood Count				
RBC	(F) 3.9–4.5 (M) 4.2–4.9			
HgB	(F) 13.5–14.5 (M) 14.0–15.0			
Hct	(F) 37.0–44.0 (M) 40.0–48.0%			
MCV	82–89.9			
MCH	27.0–31.9%			
WBC	5,000–7,500			
Neutrophils	40–60%			
Lymphocytes	24–44%			
Monocytes	0–7%			
Eosinophiols	0–3%			
Basophils	0–1%			

Lab Findings Form *(Page 2 of 2)*

Lab Tests

Name: _____ **Lab Sheet #:** _____

Date:				
Calcium & Phosphorus				
Calcium	9.4–10.0				
Phosphorous	3.0–4.0				
Ca/P Ratio	~2.4				
Blood Fats				
Cholesterol	150–220				
LDL	120 or less				
HDL	(F) >60 (M) >55				
Triglycerides	70–110				
Thyroid				
T-3 Uptake	27–37%				
T3 RIA (Total T3)	100–230				
T-4 (Thyroxine)	6–12				
T7 (FTI)	same as lab norms				
TSH	2.0-4.4				
Liver & Gall Bladder				
LDH	140–200				
Alkaline Phosphatase	70–100				
SGOT (AST)	10–30				
SGPT (ALT)	10–30				
GGTP	10–30				
Total Bilirubin	0.1-1.2				

The Big Picture

It's easy to get lost in all the numbers that fill up the pages of your lab results. If you've ever been shown the reports when a doctor has given you the interpretation of your lab results, you know it can look like a completely different language.

This workbook helps you learn the basic vocabulary and how to look at the patterns of your blood work from a functional medicine perspective. This perspective lets you view your lab results in a way your doctor may not.

You may see findings in your lab work which are outside optimal range, while your doctor may be telling you the lab findings are perfectly normal. Neither of you is wrong. Your doctor is evaluating your lab findings for the presence or indications of disease; you're interested in determining body function.

You will understand the overall and fundamental functions of your body by looking at the following areas:

Primary Body Functions	
Area of Function	**Notes**
Hydration	• Water is absolutely critical to your body functions.
Electrolytes	• Salts must be present and balanced.
Energy	• Your cells must be able to make energy.
Protein	• Without digestion you can't get what your body needs in order to live. • You must have proteins to repair, maintain and regulate your body.
Blood Count	• Red blood cells carry oxygen to the cells of your body. • White blood cells give resistance to infection.
Calcium and Phosphorus	• These are like thermostats for your metabolism. • They regulate cellular processes.
Blood Fats	• These carry fuel for energy and storage. • Make hormones and regulate immune system. • Needed for the nervous system to function.
Thyroid	• Regulates metabolism.
Liver and Gall Bladder	• The liver has about 200 different functions in your body, i.e., hormones, proteins, energy, detoxification. • The gall bladder (and/or bile ducts) detoxify your system and aid digestion.

Hydration

Hydration is critical to your health. Chronic dehydration is a common underlying cause for many health problems including allergies, arthritis, ulcers, headaches, chronic fatigue, high blood pressure, low blood pressure, digestive problems, constipation, depression, joint and muscle pain, asthma, and many more.

Aside from oxygen, every other nutrient is less important than water. Drink good-quality water and a lot of it. Distilled water is by far the best.

Drink at least as many ounces of water every as are day equal to half your body weight in pounds, i.e., body weight 150 lbs. = 75 ounces water a day. (See The Elements of Health: Water.) Use more water in hot weather and with heavy exercise.

You'll know you're drinking enough water when you urine is essentially clear. Getting your urine completely clear when you're taking vitamins might be hard, because Vitamin B2 (riboflavin) tends to make your urine a very bright yellow color. But if you're drinking enough water, your urine should be clear at least some of the day.

Here's what to look for in your blood work to indicate you're dehydrated:

Dehydration	
Lab Test	**Lab Finding**
• Blood Urea Nitrogen (BUN)	Increased
• Serum Chloride	Increased
• Potassium	Increased
• Serum Creatinine	Increased
• Albumin	Increased
• Hemoglobin (HgB)	Increased
• Hematocrit (Hct)	Increased

Electrolytes

Your body needs electrical charge to function. If there is no difference in electrical charge between different parts of your body (for instance, the inside and outside of a cell membrane) no energy is produced — no production of energy, no metabolism, no nerve conduction, no muscle contraction, no transport of nutrients into the cells of your body, and no transport of wastes outside of the cell — no life! Without the charge created by electrolytes, you're dead!

Without proper electrolyte regulation, your body is in big trouble. You can identify imbalances in the regulation of your electrolytes by checking the lab results for magnesium, potassium, sodium, and chloride.

One of the best and most basic things you can do for yourself to balance electrolytes is to use natural salt (Celtic Salt), and avoid processed salt and refined foods high in processed salt.

Electrolyte Balance

Test	Result	Meaning
Magnesium	More than 2.5	• Kidney dysfunction (drink more water and Renal plus (BRC): 2-4 tablets BID or TID). • <u>Low Thyroid</u> • <u>Low Adrenal</u> • Too much antacid use.
	Less than 2.0 (Alarm range < 1.2)	• Magnesium deficiency–Mg-Zyme (BRC); see dosage in <u>Appendices: Using Supplements To Balance Body Functions: Mg-Zyme</u>.
Potassium	More than 4.5 (Alarm range > 6.0)	• <u>Low Adrenal</u> • Kidney dysfunction. Drink more water and Renal plus (BRC): 2-4 tablets BID or TID.
	Less than 4.0 (Alarm range < 3.0)	• <u>High Adrenal</u> • Diarrhea • Use of prescription diuretics.
Sodium	More than 142 (Alarm range > 150)	• <u>Dehydration</u> • <u>High Adrenal</u> • Use of water softeners. • Kidney dysfunction (as above). • Too much salt in diet (usually commercial).
	Less than 135 (Alarm range < 128)	• <u>Low Adrenal</u> • Diarrhea • Diabetes. See <u>Using Lab Tests: Energy</u>. • Kidney dysfunction (as above). • Excessive perspiration or salt-restricted diet.
Chloride	More than 106 (Alarm range > 112)	• Kidney dysfunction (as above). • Low carbon dioxide (CO_2). See <u>Using Lab Tests: Energy</u>. • Use of aspirin and related medications. • Excessive salt use (usually commercial). • <u>High Adrenal</u> • <u>Dehydration</u>
	Less than 100 (Alarm range < 92)	• Kidney dysfunction (as above). • High carbon dioxide (CO_2). Consult physician if breathing problems are present; drink more water, Renal plus (BRC): 2-4 tablets BID or TID. • <u>Low Adrenal</u> • Breathing problems (consult physician).

> greater than   < less than

Energy (Glucose and CO_2)

These organelles turn glucose — derived from carbohydrates, fats, and proteins — into a molecule called ATP. ATP molecules provide energy to make every vital system and process function. Without ATP, you die. With too little, you just feel like you'd rather die. Common symptoms of this system not working properly are fatigue, irritability, joint and muscle aches and pain, headaches, no endurance, always sleepy, inability to concentrate, and anxiety.

Check Glucose and CO_2 values to determine your ability to make energy. The most common and early sign of impaired energy production is low CO_2.

Balancing Energy

Test	Result	Meaning
Glucose	More than 95 (Alarm range > 160)	• Diabetes — see Glycated Hemoglobin below. • Insulin Resistance. See Blood Fats. • Vitamin B Deficiency.
	Less than 80 (Alarm range < 50)	• Hypoglycemia — Blood Sugar Problems. • Low Adrenal.
Glycated Hemoglobin*	More than 7	• A high glycated hemoglobin confirms diabetes and indicates the need to work with a physician. • Often solving insulin resistance (See Using Lab Tests: Blood Fats) will clear Type II/adult onset diabetes or at least lead to better management.
	Less than 7	• Normal.
CO2	More than 31 (Alarm range > 36)	• Breathing problems — consult a physician. • Kidney dysfunction — more water and Renal plus (BRC) 2-4 tablets BID or TID.
	Less than 26 (Alarm range < 18)	• Vitamin B deficiency is the most common cause of low CO_2. • Kidney dysfunction — drink more water and Renal plus (BRC): 2-4 tablets BID or TID. • Diabetes — See Glycated Hemoglobin above to confirm. • Dehydration.

> greater than   < less than

* Glycated hemoglobin isn't a part of the standard lab panel. I've included it here because it is the best test to determine whether or not you have diabetes and for tracking the results of care.

Note: Low CO_2 is most commonly due to a Vitamin B Deficiency.

The flowchart below guides you in balancing your ability to make energy at the cellular level. The flowchart below is magic. It will often help you solve chronic fatigue when nothing else has worked.

Low CO_2

Fatigue, irritability, joint and muscle aches and pains, headaches, no endurance, always sleepy, inability to concentrate, anxiety.

Take natural Vitamin B
Bio-3BG (BRC) or Nutritional Yeast (KAL)

Symptoms resolve temporarily, then return.
Add:
Phosphorus
Without response, add:
Coenzyme Q10 (CoQ10)

No response to natural Vitamin B.
Add:
Manganese
Without response add:
Lipoic acid

Restoring Cell Energy Production

Deficiency	Supplement		Notes
Natural Vitamin B	Bio-3BG (BRC)	6 tablets TID for one bottle 6 tablets BID for one bottle 3-6 tablets a day thereafter	Chew the tablets for best response; can be taken with food.
	Nutritional Yeast	2 heaping Tbsp in water or dilute juice (grapefruit best) once or twice a day. *Note:* Must be KAL brand Nutritional Yeast.	Best source of B vitamins in natural form; though inconvenient and not always tolerated.
Phosphorus	Liquid Phosphozyme (BRC)	10-30 drops BID or TID in water.	Decreases stiffness.
	Lecithin (BRC/generic)	2-3 perles BID or TID	Decreases stiffness.
CoQ10	CoQ30 (BRC)	1-2 tablets BID	Increases oxygen saturation of body.
Manganese	MN-Zyme forte (BRC)	1-2 tablets BID	Strengthens joints.
Lipoic Acid	Lipoic acid capsules (generic/BRC)	1-2 capsules BID or TID	Possible mercury toxicity.*

* If your energy increases when using lipoic acid, you may have mercury toxicity. Get tested for mercury levels with a hair analysis (available from *The Elements of Health*). If levels are above normal, consult a physician (preferably one practicing functional medicine).

Protein

Your body can't repair and maintain itself without proteins. It's a lot like only putting gas into a car. That car will run for a while, but without getting the oil changed and parts replaced, it's going to start falling apart.

Enzymes, hormones, muscles, neurotransmitters (nerve chemicals), bones, connective tissues, every cell in your body is made up of protein. Most people are protein-deficient. It seems strange when we eat so much protein. The problem is that most of the protein we typically eat is cooked.

When proteins are cooked, some of the essential amino acids are broken down and aren't available for our bodies to use for making protein. Essential amino acids are exactly that, essential. When you have the essential amino acids, your body can make any other amino acid and any protein it needs. A lot of the various things people suffer from when they get older are a result of their bodies being protein-deficient; the vital parts aren't getting repaired or replaced.

Getting more protein (especially more raw protein) in your diet makes a profound difference in your health. See The Elements of Health: Foundation Diet.

Protein or Amino Acid Deficiency

Test	Result	Alarm Range	Meaning
BUN	Less than 10	< 6.0	Protein deficiency
Calcium	Less than 9.4	< 7.0	Protein deficiency
Total Protein	More than 7.4	> 8.2	Amino acid deficiency (need for uncooked protein)
	Less than 6.9	< 6.0	Protein deficiency
Albumin	Less than 4.0	< 3.6	Protein deficiency
Globulin	More than 2.8	> 3.5	Protein deficiency due to poor digestion
	Less than 2.4	< 2.0	Protein deficiency due to poor digestion
WBC	Less than 5.0	< 3.0	Protein deficiency
Hemoglobin	Less than 13.5 (F) Less than 14 (M)	<11.0	Protein deficiency
Hematocrit	Less than 37 (F) Less than 40 (M)	< 33.0	Protein deficiency

> greater than   < less than; M = male, F = female

Solutions for Protein Deficiencies

Outcome	What to Do
Protein deficiency	• Use the Insulin Resistance Diet *(page 155).* (See Using Lab Tests: Blood Fats.) • Eat more uncooked protein. (See The Elements of Health: Foundation Diet.) • Gamoctapro (BRC): 2 Tbsp BID or TID between meals.
Amino acid deficiency	• Use the Insulin Resistance Diet *(page 155).* • Eat more uncooked protein (Foundation Diet); Amino Sport (BRC) or generic amino acid complex: 3-6 capsules BID or TID.
Protein deficiency because of poor digestion	• Digestion Problems

Blood Count (Red and White Blood Cells)

Red blood cells carry oxygen to every part of your body. White blood cells clean house and fight infection; they are scavengers scooping up and carrying away proteins, wastes, bacteria, viruses, etc. They're like the cop on the beat looking for troublemakers and making sure they don't do any harm.

Red Blood Count Appraisal

Test	Result	Meaning
Red Blood Count (RBC)	More than 4.9 (male) More than 4.5 (female) Male alarm range > 6.0 Female alarm range > 5.0	• Asthma • Emphysema
	Less than 4.2 (male) Less than 3.9 (female) Male alarm range < 3.8 Female alarm range < 3.6	• Iron-deficiency anemia
Hemoglobin (HGB)	More than 15 (male) More than 14.5 (female) Male alarm range > 17 Female alarm range >17	• Dehydration • Asthma • Emphysema
	Less than 14 (male) Less than 13.5 (female) Male alarm range < 10 Female alarm range < 10	• Iron-deficiency anemia

(continued)

Red Blood Count Appraisal *(continued)*

Test	Result	Meaning
Hematocrit	More than 48 (male) More than 44 (female) Alarm range > 54	• Dehydration • Asthma • Emphysema
	Less than 40 (male) Less than 37 (female) Alarm range < 34	• Iron-deficiency anemia
MCV Anemia	More than 89.9 Alarm range > 95	• Vitamin B12/Folic Acid
	Less than 82.0 Alarm range < 78	• Iron-deficiency anemia • Vitamin B6 anemia • Heavy-metal toxicity
MCH anemia	More than 31.9 Alarm range > 34.0	• Vitamin B12/Folic Acid
	Less than 28.0 Alarm range < 24.0	• Iron-deficiency anemia • Vitamin B6 anemia • Heavy-metal toxicity

> greater than   < less than

Red Blood Count Outcome and Recommendations

Outcome	Possible Causes and What to Do
Asthma	• Low Adrenal • Allergies • Fatty Acids Deficiency
Emphysema	• Protein deficiency (See Using Lab Tests: Protein) • Vitamin C with bioflavinoids (generic/BRC): 4-6 grams a day. • Sulfur MSM Plus (BRC): 2-6 caps a day.
Iron-deficient anemia	• Digestion Problems • Fe-Zyme (BRC): 1 tab TID.
Vitamin B12/ Folic acid anemia	• B-12 2000 (BRC): 1 TID between meals. • Folic Acid 800 (BRC): 1 TID with meals.
Vitamin B6 anemia	• B6 Phosphate (BRC): 1-2 tablets TID with meals.
Heavy-metal toxicity	• Get a Hair Analysis. (See Using Lab Tests: Specialty Tests to Consider.) • If heavy-metal toxicity is present, consult a physician (preferably one practicing functional medicine).

White Blood Count Appraisal

Test	Result	Alarm Range	Meaning
White Blood Count (RBC)	More than 7,500	> 13,000	• Acute bacterial or viral infection
	Less than 5,000	< 3,500	• Chronic viral or bacterial infection
Neutrophils	More than 60	> 80	• Acute bacterial or viral infection
	Less than 40	< 30	• Chronic viral or bacterial infection
Lymphocytes	More than 44	> 52	• Chronic viral (maybe bacterial) infection
	Less than 24	< 20	• Acute viral or bacterial infection
Monocytes	More than 7	>14	• Inflammation somewhere in the body • Recovery stage of infection • Intestinal infections
Eosinophils	More than 3		• Intestinal infections • Allergies
Basophils	More than 1		• Inflammation • Intestinal infections

> greater than   < less than

White Blood Count Outcome and Recommendations

Outcome	What To do
Acute infection	• Echinacea Tincture (generic): 40 drops per hour decreasing to QID as symptoms improve. • Vitamin C (generic): up 10 grams a day (decrease dosage if stools are loose). • Consider juice fasting for 1-2 days.
Recovery stage of infection	• Shitake Mushroom (generic/BRC): 2-4 capsules TID. • Bio-Immunozyme (BRC): 1 tablet TID with meals. • Cytozyme AD (BRC): 2 tablets TID.
Chronic infection	• Shitake Mushroom (generic/BRC): 2-4 capsules TID. • Bio-Immunozyme (BRC): 1 tablet TID with meals. • IAG (BRC): 1-2 tsp TID.
Allergies	• Allergies
Inflammation	• Intenzyme Forte (BRC): 3-4 tablets BID TID between meals (on an empty stomach).
Intestinal infections	• Stool Culture from IPD, 480-767-2522. By far the most accurate and inexpensive test for confirming or ruling out intestinal infections, including parasites • Bromelain Plus CLA (BRC): 3-4 tablets TID between meals (empty stomach) for six weeks. • ADP (BRC): 1 tab with each meal; 1 tab at bedtime.

Note: Intestinal infections are a common underlying cause in many functional and pathological illnesses. If severe gastrointestinal symptoms are present, see a physician.

Calcium and Phosphorus

These are regulators of your metabolism as a whole. They play a vital role in balancing the conscious and unconscious functions of your nervous system (autonomic nervous system), cell-membrane transport of nutrients and wastes, and production of energy.

Calcium and Phosphorus Balance

Test	Result	Meaning
Calcium	More than 10.0 (Alarm range > 10.4)	• Parathyroid dysfunction • Excess Vitamin D
	Less than 9.4 (Alarm range < 7.0)	• Osteoporosis • Parathyroid dysfunction
Phosphorus	More than 4.0 (Alarm range > 5.0)	• Normal in growing kids and when a fracture is healing • Kidney dysfunction • Parathyroid dysfunction
	Less than 3.4 (Alarm range < 2.0)	• Need for stomach enzymes (hypochlorhydria) • Protein or amino acid deficiency
Calcium/ Phosphorus	Ratio More than 2.5	• Phosphorus deficiency
	Less than 2.3	• Calcium deficiency

> greater than   < less than

Calcium and Phosphorus Outcome and Recommendations

Outcome	What To Do
Parathyroid dysfunction	• CA/MG Plus (BRC): 1-2 tablets TID.
Excess Vitamin D	• Avoid Vitamin D-fortified foods.
Osteoporosis	• Osteo-B Plus (BRC): 2 tabs TID with meals. • See Fatty Acids Deficiency. • Check Using Home Tests: Body pH. • CA/MG Plus (BRC): 1-2 tablets TID.
Kidney dysfunction	• More water. • Renal Plus (BRC): 2-4 tablets BID/TID.
Need of stomach enzymes	• See Digestion Problems.
Protein/amino acid deficiency	• See Using Lab Tests: Protein. • Refer to The Elements of Health: Foundation Diet.
Phosphorus deficiency	• See Digestion Problems. • Super Phosphozyme Liquid (BRC): 1-2 D BID.
Calcium deficiency	• Osteo-B Plus (BRC): 2 tabs TID with meals. • See The Elements of Health: Foundation Diet. • See Digestion Problems.

Blood Fats (Cholesterol, Triglycerides and HDL)

Eating a low-fat diet makes you fat, gives you diabetes, causes heart disease, and upsets the normal balance of male and female hormones resulting in menstrual problems, polycystic ovaries, and prostate disease. Eating a low-fat diet harms your nervous system and hinders your ability to produce hormones. Low-fat diets cause osteoporosis and premature aging.

Want to control your cholesterol? Want to lower your cholesterol/HDL ratio so your risk for heart disease is lower? Eat fats, eat protein, eat vegetables. The sodas, candy, and pasta are causing the trouble, not the cheese and the eggs.

High carbohydrate and low fat-diets cause insulin resistance. Here's how to determine if you have insulin resistance and what to do about it:

Insulin Resistance

Lab Test	Finding	What To Do
Glucose	More than 95 (Alarm range > 160)	• Use the Insulin Resistance Diet. • Do Aerobic Exercise 3 days a week. • Weight train 3 days a week. • Glucobalance (BRC): 2 caps TID. or Nutritional Yeast (KAL): 2 Tbsp BID. • PCOH-Plus (BRC): 1 capsule BID. • Check Fatty Acids Deficiency. • Check for High Adrenal. • See Using Lab Tests: Protein.
Cholesterol	More than 220 (Alarm range > 300)	
Low-Density Lipoproteins (LDL)	More than 120 (Alarm range > 200)	
High-Density Lipoproteins (HDL)	Less than 55 (males) Less than 60 (females) (Alarm range < 35)	
Triglycerides	More than 110 (Alarm range > 280)	

Policosanol from PCOH-Plus is proven to lower cholesterol (an average of 23% in six weeks), raise HDL, and decrease platelet aggregation (decreasing the risk of stroke and heart attack) without the toxicity associated with cholesterol-lowering medications.

> greater than   < less than

Insulin resistance means your body doesn't respond properly to insulin. Our bodies were not designed to eat the large quantity of carbohydrates found in today's typical diet. The result is an excessive and constant release of insulin. When our bodies are repeatedly bathed in insulin, our bodies will stop responding to it. The result is obesity, high cholesterol and triglycerides, diabetes, chronic fatigue (especially after eating), male and female hormone imbalances, osteoporosis, heart disease, and joint degeneration.

If you've been frustrated after trying every diet in the world and still struggle with your weight, following the diet and exercise programs for insulin resistance along with the supplements in the above table will be a godsend for you.

Insulin is the single most powerful anabolic hormone in your body. Anabolic refers to insulin's activity in repairing and maintaining your body. Your body, every part of it, starts to break down if you're not responding to insulin.

Insulin resistance accounts for a lot of the degeneration you see as people age. Much of what we typically attribute to aging isn't really because of getting older. Most of aging is actually accumulated neglect and bad habits catching up with people.

You can control your cholesterol with a low-fat diet consisting of low-fat meats and vegetables only; however, it's not a good strategy for long-term good health, because over time, deficiencies of essential fatty acids and fat-soluble nutrients will result.

Using cholesterol-lowering drugs isn't a good idea, either. Cholesterol-lowering drugs work by blocking some of your liver functions. Get your liver tested regularly if you take these drugs.

Using the Insulin Resistance Diet and getting more exercise will reverse insulin resistance. You will know it does because of how much better you feel, and because you'll see balance in your lab work. Give it time. Insulin resistance develops over a lifetime. It may take up to six months before your body really takes to the changes in diet and exercise.

Insulin Resistance Diet

- Use the Foundational Diet for general principles of diet.

- For the first two weeks, limit your carbohydrate intake (carbs) to 30 grams or less each day.

- After the first two weeks, limit your carbohydrate intake to 60 grams or less each day.

- Use a food table book to calculate the carbs you're eating each day (available at bookstores; make sure the food table includes a listing for the fiber content of each food).

- True carbs are the total carbs minus the fiber content (true carbs = total carbs — fiber).

- Zero-carb foods are cabbage, celery, broccoli, lettuce, spinach, onions, asparagus, mushrooms, peppers and radishes — you can eat these freely.

- Don't go any longer than three hours without eating (except when sleeping).

Exercise for Insulin Resistance

- Weight train full body with free weights 3 times a week.
- Use compound movements only.
- Use 4-6 reps per movement with high weight short of failure.*
- Don't work out for longer than 40 minutes.
- Eat only protein or nothing before exercise.
- Eat a protein-focused, low-fat and low-carbohydrate meal shortly after working out.
- Change your workout routine often.
- Use interval-type aerobic training 3-6 times a week.*
- Stretch every day (preferably using yoga-style stretching).
- Take one day off a week from training.
- Have fun!

Note: For more direction, refer to The Elements of Health: Exercise. Consider working with a physical trainer until you are clear about how to exercise properly.

Exercise 20-40 minutes each day. That's all it takes to turn insulin resistance around.

If you have limited time for exercise, alternate aerobic and anaerobic exercise. The following table might be useful to you in planning your exercise routine.

Monday	Tuesday	Wednesday	Thursday	Friday	Saturday	Sunday
Weight Training	Aerobic Training	Weight Training	Aerobic Training	Weight Training	Aerobic Training	Rest

Thyroid

Your thyroid controls the rate of your metabolism. It's kind of like the idle in your car — if it runs too slowly, your engine will run cold, sputter, and wheeze. If your idle is turned up too high, your engine will rev too fast and suffer from too much wear and tear.

Thyroid Function Appraisal		
Test	**Result**	**Meaning**
T3 Uptake (T3U)	More than 37 (Alarm range > 39)	• High Thyroid • Too much thyroid medication
	Less than 27 (Alarm range < 22)	• Low Thyroid • Too much estrogen medication/birth control
T3 RIA or Total T3	More than 230 (Alarm range > 240)	• High Thyroid • Too much thyroid medication
	Less than 100 (Alarm range < 70)	• Low Thyroid • Too much estrogen medication/birth control
T4	More than lab normal (Alarm range > 13.0)	• High Thyroid • Too much estrogen medication (including birth control pills)
	Less than lab normal (Alarm range < 5.0)	• Low Thyroid • Low Pituitary • Steroid use
T7 (FTI)	More than 11.0 (Alarm range > 13.0)	• High Thyroid • Too much thyroid medication
	Less than 6.0 (Alarm range < 4.8)	• Low Thyroid • Too much estrogen medication/birth control
TSH (a pituitary hormone)	More than 4.4 (Alarm range > 9.0)	• Low Thyroid
	Less than 2.0 (Alarm range < 0.3)	• High Thyroid • Low Pituitary

> greater than   < less than

High Thyroid — When T3U, Total T3, T4, and T7 (thyroid values) are high and the TSH (thyroid-stimulating hormone from the pituitary) is low, you have High Thyroid.

High Pituitary — When thyroid values are high and the TSH is high, you have High Pituitary.

Low Thyroid — When thyroid values are low and the TSH is high, you have Low Thyroid.

Low Pituitary — When thyroid values are low and the TSH is low, you have Low Pituitary.

Thyroid Outcome and Recommendations

Outcome	Possible Causes and What To Do
High Thyroid	• See <u>High Thyroid</u> and follow the recommendations.
High Pituitary	• See <u>High Pituitary</u> and follow the recommendations.
Low Thyroid	• See <u>Low Thyroid</u> and follow the recommendations.
Low Pituitary	• See <u>Low Pituitary</u> and follow the recommendations.
Excess Steroids	• If prescription, look to <u>Stress and Life</u> as restoring function to the adrenal glands may overcome the need for prescription steroids (prednisone, cortisone, etc.). Consult with your physician if you are on prescription steroids and want to restore adrenal function; you may need guidance from a physician who is knowledgeable in functional medicine. • Use the <u>Health Graph</u>, <u>Home Tests</u> and <u>Lab Tests</u> for guidance in resolving the health problem for which you're taking steroid medication. • The side-effects of steroid use for athletics and bodybuilding can't be justified in light of the long-term destruction of health.
Excess Estrogen	• It is common to be prescribed estrogen for female-related problems when the actual problem is in too much estrogen in relation to other hormones. • Birth control pills have many side-effects; use alternate birth control whenever possible. • Consider getting a female hormonal panel done to understand the balance between estrogen, testosterone, progesterone, and DHEA. (See <u>Using Lab Tests: Specialty Tests To Consider</u>.)

Liver and Gall Bladder

When you feel poorly and nothing you do helps, if your body just doesn't seem to work right, if you don't respond to any treatment, if you can't seem to make sense of all the health problems you're suffering from and don't know what to do or where to go next, focus on your liver and gall bladder.

If your lab values for liver and/or gall bladder function are outside of the reference ranges, make sure to do a cleanse (<u>The Elements of Health: Detoxification and Fasting</u>) and to support your liver and gall bladder according to <u>Health Graph: Liver/Gall Bladder</u>.

Why is it so important to do cleansing and support your liver? Today's toxic environment. In the last 100 years, thousands of toxic chemicals have been created that our bodies were never designed to deal with. This burden is making most of us sick to at least some degree, and limiting the fullest expression of our inherent health.

Liver and Gall Bladder Function

Test	Result	Meaning
LDH	More than 200 (Alarm range > 240)	• Liver dysfunction • Gall bladder/Bile duct dysfunction • Anemia • Heart dysfunction • Too much estrogen
	Less than 140 (Alarm range < 80)	• Hypoglycemia
Alkaline Phosphatase (ALP)	More than 100 (Alarm range > 130)	• Osteoporosis • Rheumatoid arthritis • Gall bladder/Bile duct dysfunction
	Less than 70 (Alarm range < 30)	• Zinc Deficiency
SGOT (AST)	More than 30 (Alarm range > 100)	• Heart disease • Liver dysfunction
	Less than 10	• Vitamin B6 Deficiency
SGPT (ALT)	More than 30 (Alarm range > 100)	• Liver dysfunction
	Less than 10	• Vitamin B6 Deficiency
GGTP (GGT)	More than 30 (Alarm range > 90)	• Gall bladder/bile duct dysfunction • Liver dysfunction • Too much alcohol • Digestive dysfunction
	Less than 10	• Vitamin B6 Deficiency
Total Bilirubin	More than 1.2 (Alarm range > 2.2)	• Liver dysfunction • Gall bladder/bile duct dysfunction • Anemia

> greater than   < less than

Note: GGTP will be higher than the SGOT (AST) and SGPT (ALT) with dysfunction of the gall bladder or bile ducts, and lower than SGOT and SGPT when liver dysfunction is the primary problem.

Liver and Gall Bladder Outcome and Recommendations

Outcome	What To Do
Liver dysfunction	• Liver/Gall Bladder • See The Elements of Health: Detoxification and Fasting.
Gall bladder/ Bile duct dysfunction	• Liver/Gall Bladder • See The Elements of Health: Detoxification and Fasting. • Avoid **all** white flour, sugar, and hydrogenated fats (especially margarine). • Lecithin (generic/BRC) *Note:* BRC's lecithin is labeled Phosphatidylcholine, 1-3 capsules BID.
Anemia	• See Using Lab Tests: Blood Count.
Heart dysfunction	• Heart Function • If liver enzymes are at or past the alarm values, heart disease is a strong possibility. If this is so, see a physician for isoenzyme studies of the liver enzymes to confirm or rule out the presence of heart disease.
Too much estrogen	• Consider a saliva female or male hormonal study to measure estrogen levels. See Using Lab Tests: Specialty Tests to Consider. • Adjust dosage or eliminate estrogen medication. • You may be sensitive to the presence of estrogen in foods (commercial animal products — meat, chicken, eggs, milk, butter, etc.); use organic animal products. • Plastics and pesticides act like estrogen in your body (xenobiotics). Avoid these in your environment. • Use soy in your diet (8 oz of soy milk a day is adequate) to bind estrogen receptors and decrease overall estrogen activity.
Hypoglycemia	• Blood Sugar Problems
Osteoporosis	• See Calcium and Phosphorus section, Using Lab Tests: Calcium and Phosphorus.
Rheumatoid arthritis	• Low Adrenal • Fatty Acids Deficiency • Liver/Gall Bladder • Digestion Problems • Using Lab Tests: Protein • See The Elements of Health: Detoxification and Fasting. • Allergies • Take a lab test called C-Reactive Protein (CRP) to monitor your progress; optimum value is less than five (<5); values should decrease as you get better.

(continued)

Liver and Gall Bladder Outcome and Recommendations *(continued)*

Outcome	What To Do
Zinc deficiency	• <u>Nutritional Deficiency</u>. • Take the <u>Zinc Taste Test</u>.
Vitamin B6 deficiency	• See <u>Nutritional Deficiency</u>.
Digestive Dysfunction	• See <u>Using Lab Tests: Protein</u>. • See <u>Digestion Problems</u>.
GGTP Higher Than Other Enzymes	• Confirms the primary problem is in the gall bladder or bile ducts.
Other Enzymes Higher Than GGTP	• Confirms a liver problem is more likely than a gall bladder or bile duct problem — if enzymes are above alarms, heart disease is possible; see a physician.

Specialty Tests To Consider

All of the following tests, including a report with findings, interpretation and recommendations, are available from Dr. Force through the *The Elements of Health*, 866-563-4256 or from doctors endorsing and incorporating the *choosing* HEALTH system with their patients.

Specialty Tests Resources

Specialty Diagnostic Laboratories

Diagnos-Techs (DT) 800-878-3787 diagnostechs.com	Great Smokies (GS) 800-522-4762 gsdl.com	Metametrix (MM) 800-221-4640 metametrix.com

Test & Lab	Sample	Function
Serum Amino Acids (MM)	Blood	• Tests for specific need for individual amino acids • Helps balance genetic weaknesses in metabolism
Adrenal Stress Index (DT) **Adrenocortex Stress Profile (GS)** **Adrenal Stress — Saliva (MM)**	Saliva	• Determines the type of <u>Adrenal Dysfunction</u> • Determines best way to balance adrenals
Expanded Female Hormonal Panel (DT) **Female Hormone (GS)**	Saliva	• Tests **all** of the female hormones over a whole menstrual cycle • Determines how to optimize female hormones
Postmenopausal Panel (DT) **Menopause Profile (GS)**	Saliva	• A panel for women who no longer menstruate

(continued)

Specialty Tests Resources (continued)

Test & Lab	Sample	Function
Male Hormonal Panel (DT) **Male Hormone Profile (GS)**	Saliva	• Tests the dynamics of male hormones. • Determines how to optimize male hormones.
Extended Gastrointestinal Panel (DT) **Comprehensive Digestive Stool Analysis (GS)**	Stool and Saliva	• Tests for digestive function, infections, and balance of healthy flora. • Tests allergies to milk, grains, soy, and eggs.
Comprehensive Food Allergies (GS)	Blood	• Tests for food allergies (both immediate and delayed-type allergic reactions). • Tests for allergies to your environment. (grasses, trees, molds, animals, dust, etc.) • Area-specific environmental allergy panels.
Elemental Analysis (GS) **Elements Hair (MM)**	Hair	• Tests for minerals and toxic metals.

Urine Amino Acid Panel (MM)

Many people have problems assimilating and utilizing amino acids properly because of their genetic makeup. This test helps determine your unique needs for certain proportions of amino acids and, from the test, a formula of amino acids can be tailored to balance your metabolism.

This test is remarkably helpful when you have balanced your protein according to your blood test but still don't feel fantastic. I also recommend this test for chronic fatigue, allergies, managing seizures, preventing cardiovascular disease, rheumatoid arthritis, Candida albicans, athletic performance, behavior disorders, learning disabilities, and improving your overall health, especially if you're older.

Adrenal Stress Index Test (DT)
Adrenocortex Stress Profile (GS)
Adrenal Stress – Saliva (MM)

This test provides DHEA levels and cortisol rhythm. Get this test done if you have found Low Adrenal or High Adrenal and when you do follow-up Health Graphs, and your adrenal function isn't changing. Also do this test when you have very chronic fatigue problems or any time the work you're doing for yourself based on the Health Graph, Home Tests, and Lab Tests doesn't make a difference.

Expanded Female Hormonal Panel (DT)
Female Hormone (GS)

Blood tests are not an accurate way to determine hormone levels. Though it is still very common for doctors to use blood tests for hormones, saliva is considered the standard in a research setting. Balancing female hormone problems is complicated at best; if your hormones don't respond to working with the health appraisal, home tests, and lab interpretation, get a female hormone panel to sort out the pattern.

This panel tests for three estrogens (estriol, estradiol, and estrone), progesterone, testosterone, DHEA, follicle-stimulating hormone (FSH), and luteinizing hormone (LH). This test also takes 11 measurements of estrogen and progesterone through one menstrual cycle to determine the dynamics of hormones during your menstrual cycle. By getting the whole picture of hormones, you can get to the bottom of what is going on.

Expanded Post-Menopausal Hormonal Panel (DT)
Menopausal Profile (GS)

This is the panel for female hormones when a woman is no longer menstruating.

Expanded Male Hormonal Panel (DT)
Male Hormone Profile (GS)

Male hormones are much more than just testosterone. Do you convert too much of your testosterone to estrogen? The ratio of testosterone to estrogen is just as important to your male characteristics as the total amount of testosterone in your body.

Is too much of your testosterone being converted into DHT, increasing your risk for prostate cancer? Do you have enough DHEA and androstenedione to make testosterone? Does your pituitary release enough of the hormones LH and FSH for your body to make adequate testosterone?

Expanded Gastrointestinal Health Panel (DT)
Comprehensive Digestive Stool Analysis (GS)

Run this test if you have already done a couple of Health Appraisals and lab interpretations and you're still having digestive problems, or if the digestive problems are chronic. This panel is also used to determine if any infections are present in your digestive tract.

Comprehensive Antibody Assessment (GS)

If you test very high in the Allergies section of the Health Graph and/or your Eosinophils are high when checking the Blood Count section of Using Lab Tests, you may want to get this test done. This panel is very useful on finding delayed allergic reactions. Delayed reactions (IGG-mediated) can't be tested with the traditional scratch testing done on the skin by most allergists.

This test screens you for 96 of the most common food allergens and grades the severity of any positive allergic reactions.

Common symptoms of hidden food allergies are fatigue, joint and muscle stiffness and pain, headaches, feeling foggy-headed, anxiety, poor sleep, waking up tired, and weight gain or inability to lose weight. I have seen people transformed by getting allergic foods out of their diet.

Great Smokies Diagnostic Laboratory (GS) has panels for inhalant allergens (dust, grasses, trees, molds, etc.) specific for different regions of the country. This enables you to be tested for the particular allergens you're exposed to in your area.

It is now possible to make homeopathic formulas specific to the allergens to which you're sensitive. My experience has been that using homeopathy to desensitize you for inhalant allergens tends to be quicker, less expensive, and much more simpler than traditional approaches (injections).

Elemental Analysis (GS)
Elements Hair (MM)
Hair Elements (DD)
Hair analysis is useful to determine trace mineral need and problems from toxic metals.

Stress is a term originally coined by Hans Selye, MD, a pioneer of stress research in the 1930s. He authored several hundred papers as well as two landmark books on the topic: *The Stress Of Life* and *Stress Without Distress*. Since then, related research has confirmed his theories.

As a teenager, Dr. Selye's theories gave me the answers I needed to recover from colitis, chronic infections, and allergies. Once I'd read *The Stress Of Life*, I understood how stress was the cause of most disease. It is the missing element for many people who have searched and researched for answers regarding their health problems, only to be told that no answers existed for their illness; they would just have to tough it out and learn to live with it.

It's a word we often use to describe our busy, event-packed lives, but what does the term *stress* really mean? Mostly, we think of emotional stress, but there are actually four types: emotional, physical, chemical, and thermal.

What is Stress?

According to Dr. Selye, stress is any stimulus to your system (body) that requires it to respond or adapt. Normally, your body adapts to stress and maintains a healthy and balanced state called homeostasis.

A stressor is anything that causes stress. Dr. Selye categorized stressors by the manner in which they cause stress. There are four types according to Selye: physical (mechanical), chemical, thermal, and emotional.

We can handle and adapt to only so much stress before something starts to give. Using an analogy, our life can be compared to a bucket. Once our bucket is filled to the brim with stress, the excess spills over and manifests as symptoms, all because our ability to adapt has been overwhelmed.

Everyone has a different-sized bucket based on their inherent strengths and weaknesses. If your bucket becomes too full, you're in trouble. We could argue it was the last drop of water that started the problem, but, at some point — preferably *before* your bucket spills over — have the foresight to pour off enough water to prevent an overflow. Each time you face a health problem, ask yourself: "How much do I need to spill from my bucket in order for my body to be able to handle the remainder of my life and heal?"

On the following page is a brief list of examples for each of the four types of stress according to Dr. Selye.

Four Types of Stress

Physical (Mechanical)
- Inadequate sleep or rest
- Inadequate work/exercise
- Repetitive or asymmetrical movement at work/play
- Physical injuries
- Excessive or imbalanced work/exercise
- Unsupportive furniture, shoes, beds, etc.

Chemical
- Air and/or water pollution
- Pesticides and herbicides, solvents, industrial chemicals
- Flavorings, colorings, and preservatives
- Refined foods (hydrogenated oils, white flour, sugar)
- Antibiotics (and medications, in general)
- Dental amalgam (fillings)

Mental
- Poor relationships and financial burdens
- Past emotional trauma
- Self judgments (especially self-expectations of perfection)
- Anticipation of harm, pain, or dreaded events

Thermal
- Extreme or prolonged heat or cold
- Extreme changes in temperature

I have studied and used Dr. Selye's work for many years. I propose that your body responds to thermal stress through changes in your body's chemistry. So although the agent of the stress may be thermal, the response to that stressor is mediated through your body's chemical processes.

By extension of this thinking, there are four types of agents which cause stress, but there are only three ways your body responds; through chemical, physical, or mental processes. These processes represent the Triad of Health and are the three aspects that control your health.

Distress and the Adrenal Glands

Dr. Selye found that your body reacts to anything stressful in exactly the same way, regardless of the type of stressor involved. Ironically, he discovered that situations — both good and bad — can cause stress.

He found that some forms of stress are not necessarily bad for you. Although severe, prolonged stress (distress) always results in disease, mild and intermittent stress (eustress) actually tends to make the body healthier. A good example of eustress is exercise followed by rest.

Prolonged distress always results in abnormal function of the adrenal glands which are located above each kidney. They release hormones to help your body adapt to stress. Following are the four main groups of hormones manufactured by the adrenal glands.

Adrenal Hormones

Mineralcorticoids

These control the balance of electrolytes in your body. Electrolyte balance controls nerve function, muscle function, transport of nutrients into every cell of your body (and waste products out), and even the chemical processes of metabolism.

Glucocorticoids

These hormones regulate your blood sugar, control the maintenance, repair, and regeneration of every cell of your body, regulate your immune system, and act as antiinflammatory agents (control inflammation). The primary glucocorticoid is cortisol.

Sexual Corticoids

The adrenal glands account for about 15% of a male's testosterone; for females, it is significantly higher. Testosterone increases muscle mass, bone density, rate of metabolism, libido, and blood count. Though the amount of estrogens produced by the adrenal glands is relatively small, it is enough to control the symptoms of menopause and prevent osteoporosis.

Catecholamine

Adrenaline (epinephrine) and noradrenaline (norepinephrine) stimulate the nervous system and trigger the fight-or-flight response (sympathetic nervous system). The fight-or-flight response is characterized by increased heart rate and blood pressure, increased nerve and muscle tone (resulting in nervousness and muscle spasms), pupil dilation, and cold, clammy skin (especially of hands and feet). The functions of your digestive tract also shut down, resulting in all kinds of digestion problems which commonly include constipation, gas, bloating, irritable bowel syndrome, diverticulitis, and colitis. Production of hormones from the thyroid and testes/ovaries decrease from the influence of catecholamines.

General Adaptive Syndrome

The General Adaptive Syndrome (GAS) is a phenomenon originally observed by Dr. Selye. It represents the changes in the levels of hormones produced by the adrenal glands in response to prolonged stress.

There are three stages to the General Adaptive Syndrome (GAS):

- **Alarm**
- **Resistance**
- **Exhaustion**

The Alarm Stage represents your initial response to stress. Initially, you don't produce enough adrenal hormones for your body to adapt.

General Adaptive Syndrome

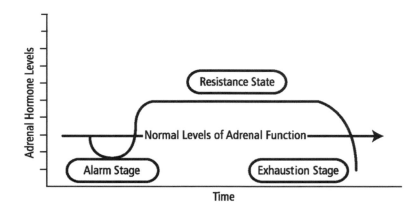

In the Resistance Stage, your adrenal glands produce more than normal amounts of adrenal hormones so your body can adapt to the excessive demands being made upon it. The adrenal glands actually become larger at this point. Output of adrenal hormones at this stage is greater than normal, and the reserves of the system overall are being drained.

The Exhaustion Stage is the point where the body's ability to adapt has been exhausted, and symptoms and illness result. Adrenal hormone levels decline and every part of your body, even at the cellular level, is markedly compromised. I would estimate from clinical experience that at least 70% of chronic and degenerative diseases are at least complicated, if not caused, by people being in the exhaustion phase of the General Adaptive Syndrome. At this stage, people tend to respond slowly to healing. It's much like when a battery is completely drained — it takes time to recharge.

Later in this section, you will learn how to determine what stage of the GAS your body is in. This is a powerful tool, because it gives you more detailed direction and greater insight into restoring adrenal function than the general recommendations in High Adrenal and Low Adrenal from the Health Graph.

Generally, when people are in the Resistance Stage, they think they're fine because they're still adapting and still able to function. It's much like having enough money in your bank account to pay the bills in the short term, but gradually paying out more than you're putting in. You can meet your needs for a while, but it won't last forever.

Being in the Resistance Stage is like that. Even though you'll get through the day and get everything done, the cost of being in this stage is high. Problems commonly include lowered resistance to infection, high blood pressure, osteoporosis, muscle atrophy, increased body fat, high cholesterol, arteriosclerosis (heart disease), nervousness, anxiety, depression, and insomnia.

The Results of Stress on Body Function

Chronic stress affects not only the overall levels of adrenal hormones, it also alters the circadian rhythm of hormones released throughout the day. The integration of this day/night cycle of hormones is profoundly important to your health. Hormones work in cycles and in rhythm with one another. Many of the hormones in your body work in antagonistic ways and must be released at different times to be effective.

People who are able to reset their circadian rhythms to match their work/sleep cycle rather than the day/night cycle can remain healthy. Many don't, and their health suffers.

Cortisol, the adrenal hormone most profoundly influenced by stress, is normally released in a cycle, with the highest value being in the morning and lowest at night. When the cortisol rhythm is disrupted, energy won't be available to you when you need it during the day. And when you're asleep at night, your body won't be repairing itself.

Cortisol Rhythm

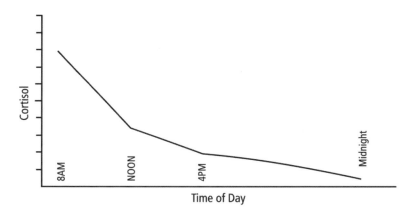

This graph illustrates cortisol's normal pattern. The left side represents the early morning (around 8 AM) and the right side represents the late evening (around 11 PM).

Low cortisol allows your body to repair and regenerate itself while you're asleep. If cortisol remains high, you may be able to sleep, but your body doesn't recharge or rebuild. If that pattern continues, things will eventually start to break down.

When the body is able to rebuild during sleep, cortisol will be high upon waking. You will feel recharged and ready to take on the world. If you wake up tired, a low morning cortisol probably has you dragging out of bed.

Under stress, cortisol levels can run very high. Abnormal circadian rhythm normally will not develop until stress is prolonged — usually over years — but it can also occur in just a few months, especially if it is severe and constant.

When the cortisol rhythm stays out of balance, more serious problems can appear, such as arthritis, allergies, asthma, colitis, ulcers, recurrent and prolonged infections, auto-immune diseases, and degeneration of the nervous system.

Effects of Abnormal Cortisol Rhythm

System	Effect
Production of Energy	Blood sugar levels and the ability of your cells to make energy are compromised. Insulin resistance results in excess body fat, diabetes, and heart disease.
Sleep	The rapid eye movement stage (REM) of the sleep cycle is interrupted by high cortisol values at night. Since REM is the most regenerative stage of sleep, fatigue, depression, and lack of mental acuity can result.
Brain	Excessive cortisol levels actually damage neurons and receptors in your brain. This probably accounts for the problems with depression, learning, and memory observed in people who are chronically stressed.
Muscle and Connective Tissues (Tendons, Ligaments and Joints)	Reduced tissue repair, coupled with an increased rate of tissue breakdown (a normal part of body metabolism), leads to an increased risk for muscle and joint injury. The lowered rate of repair and increased breakdown prevents normal repair of injuries, even everyday wear-and-tear, and leads to chronic injuries and chronic pain.
Bone	If the night cortisol is elevated, your bones do not rebuild during sleep and you are more prone to osteoporosis.
Immune System	High cortisol levels decrease the production of white blood cells. High cortisol levels decrease, immune response in the linings of the lungs, throat, kidneys, bladder, and intestinal tract. This results in lowered resistance to infection and increased risk for allergies.
Skin Regeneration	Thin, dry (even crepe-paper-like) skin is usually the result of high night cortisol levels. Human skin regenerates mostly during the night while you're asleep. Skin having moisture and resilience is a sign of healthy cortisol rhythm.
Thyroid Function	High cortisol levels inhibit thyroid hormone levels and result in fatigue, low body temperature, and weight gain.
Pituitary Gland	High cortisol levels inhibit pituitary hormone levels, affecting thyroid, male and female hormones, growth hormone levels increasing the rate of aging, and further compromising the adrenal function.
Liver	Abnormal cortisol levels stress detoxification pathways in your liver and may compromise the ability of your liver to function properly.
Intestines	Abnormal cortisol levels weaken the intestinal wall, resulting in ulcers, colitis, Crohn's Disease, Irritable Bowel Syndrome, abnormal gut flora, and Candida.

Signs and Symptoms of Adrenal Dysfunction

Because the adrenals are so important to functions throughout your body, the symptoms caused by them not functioning well can be virtually anything anywhere. Your symptoms will depend upon the pattern, chronicity, and severity of the stress you have experienced, and the nature of your inherent genetic strengths and weaknesses.

Signs and Symptoms of Adrenal Dysfunction	
Bold type = particularly common	
System	**Signs and Symptoms**
General	Fatigue, headaches (including migraines), blurred vision, anxiety, depression, weight gain, insomnia.
Neurological	Learning disabilities, Attention Deficit Disorder (ADD), insomnia, **wake tired in the morning, poor short-term and/or long term memory**, short attention span, **poor mental acuity, inability to concentrate**, dizziness when changing positions.
Immune System	**Allergies**, recurrent and/or long-lasting infections, autoimmune disorders, eczema, psoriasis.
Connective Tissue	**Dry and/or thin skin**, joint pain (especially in the low back, knees, and pelvis), lax and easily injured joints, creaking joints, tired feet, and weak ankles.
Blood Sugar	**Fatigue**, fainting spells, waking during the night, mood swings, craving sweets, sodas and/or coffee, irritability and/or shakiness before meals.
Energy Metabolism	Fatigue, low body temperature, fatigue made worse with exercise, Fluid Balance Intercellular edema (worse at mense), high or low blood pressure, dehydration, **excessive urination (15-20 times a day)**, excessive perspiration, non-pitting edema, salt cravngs.
Electrolyte Balance	Impaired nerve conduction and muscle function, heart palpitations and arrhythmias, muscle twitching, **discomfort with bright light**, sore calves, hemorrhoids, varicose veins.
Inflammatory	**Chronic upper-respiratory infections, asthma, allergies, hay fever**, skin rashes, colitis, diverticulitis, bursitis, sinusitis, enteritis, gastric-duodenal ulcers, rheumatoid arthritis, joint pain, and hives.
Hormonal	Impotence, difficulty maintaining erection, lack of genital sensitivity for female, **lack of libido in male and female**, postpartum depression, **menopausal problems, difficult and/or irregular menstrual periods.**

Note: This is a list of the possible symptoms, and not all symptoms will be present for people who have adrenal dysfunction.

How Do Your Adrenal Glands Function?

To be able to get where you want to go, you first have to figure out where you are. Do you have Adrenal Dysfunction, or do your adrenal glands function normally?

There is a very logical and clear method you can use yourself at home to determine where you stand. By doing and charting the tests outlined below, you will be able to determine precisely where you are in the General Adaptive Syndrome (GAS).

In addition to the tests we've already covered, you will need to do a Paradoxical Pupil Dilation Test to check your adrenal function. This involves shining a flashlight in one eye while looking in a mirror. Normally, your pupil should constrict and stay constricted for 30 seconds.

Paradoxical pupil dilation is present when:
- Your pupil initially constricts, but then fluctuates rhythmically.
- Your pupil initially constricts, but then dilates.
- Your pupil fluctuates by opening and closing rhythmically.
- Your pupil dilates instead of constricting to light.

Determining Your Position in the GAS			
Test	**Resistance**	**Early Exhaustion**	**Late Exhaustion**
Blood Pressure	Diastolic high	Diastolic low	Systolic and diastolic both low
Blood Pressure Dynamics	Systolic blood pressure increases more than 10mmHg when testing from lying to standing.	Systolic blood pressure usually drops when going from lying to standing; the drop may be considerable.	Systolic blood pressure usually changes little or drops from lying to standing.
Urine Sodium (norm 18-22)	Low	High	Low
Pupil Light Reaction	Constricted pupil	Paradoxical pupil dilation	Paradoxical pupil dilation

If you haven't already done so, you'll need to read the Using Home Tests section so you can take your blood pressure and run the urine sodium test.

Restoring Adrenal Function

The process of restoring adrenal function can be complex. If the problem is very chronic, it is essential you monitor your progress periodically so you can alter the approach you're using in accord with how your body is recovering. If you don't retest yourself as you go along, you'll likely reach a plateau.

There are several things you need to take care of regardless of what stage of the General Adaptive Syndrome you're in. This is the foundation of restoring adrenal function.

General Guidelines for Restoring Adrenal Function

Decrease stress	• Sleep eight (or more) hours a night. • See The Elements of Health: Breathing. • See The Elements of Health: Contemplation, Meditation, and Prayer. (Use Alternate-Nostril Breathing).
Balance the autonomic nervous system	• Check High Autonomic and Low Autonomic. • Check for Vitamin B Deficiency and Vitamin G Deficiency.
Balance your blood sugar	• See the Insulin Resistance Diet. (Using Lab Tests: Blood Fats). • See Blood Sugar Problems. • Check Using Lab Tests: Energy.
Balance antioxidants	• Run the Oxidation Stress Test. (See Using Home Tests: The Oxidation Stress Test.)
Avoid stimulants	• Cigarettes, coffee, sodas, candy, sweets in general.
Avoid drugs	• Alcohol • Recreational drugs (especially marijuana). • Over-the-counter and prescription medications.
Balance zinc	• Check the Zinc Taste Test. (Using Lab Tests: The Zinc Taste Test.) Support accordingly. Zinc decreases cortisol.
Avoid allergens	• Check Allergies and Immune System. • Consider a Comprehensive Antibody Assessment for food allergies. (Using Lab Tests: Specialty Tests to Consider.) Food allergies are a very common primary stressor causing Adrenal Dysfunction.
Avoid toxins	• Avoid hydrogenated oils, artificial sweeteners, flavorings, colorings, preservatives, solvents, air pollution, etc. • Look to The Elements of Health section for Foundation Diet and Non-Toxic Environment.

Specific Guidelines for Restoring Adrenal Dysfunction

Stage	What To Do
Resistance	<ul><li>See <u>High Pituitary</u>.</li><li>See <u>High Adrenal</u>.</li><li>Avoid commercial salt; use Celtic salt moderately.</li><li>ADHS (BRC): 2 tabs BID.</li><li>Liquid DMAE-H3 (generic; preferably made by TwinLab): 1ml in dilute juice BID.</li><li>Parasympa (DR): 2D TID for at least 6 weeks.</li><li>Exercise: All exercise recommended.*</li></ul>
Early Exhaustion	<ul><li>Use lots of Celtic salt.</li><li>ADHS (BRC): 2 tabs BID.</li><li>Parasympa (DR): 2D TID for at least 6 weeks.</li><li>Liquid DMAE-H3 (generic; preferably made by TwinLab): 1ml in dilute juice BID.</li><li>Sumacazon (AHC): 2D TID.</li><li>Exercise: Very light <u>Aerobic</u> and <u>Energetic Exercise</u>; weight train up to three times per week.*</li></ul>
Late Exhaustion	<ul><li>See <u>Low Pituitary</u>.</li><li>Parasympa (DR): 2D TID for at least 6 weeks.</li><li>Sumacazon (AHC): 2D TID.</li><li>Liquid DMAE-H3 (generic; preferably made by TwinLab): 1ml in dilute juice BID.</li><li>Cytozyme AD (BRC): 1-4 tabs TID; chewed.</li><li>Licorice Root (generic): 2-4 caps BID in the morning and at noon; decrease or discontinue as blood pressure normalizes.</li><li>Progesterone cream (generic); women take as directed; men take ¼–½ tsp a day rubbed into your skin where it is naturally thinner: inner arms and thighs, abdomen, chest and face; decrease as adrenal function improves.</li><li>Use lots of <u>Celtic Salt</u>.</li><li>Exercise: Very light <u>Aerobic</u> and <u>Energetic Exercise</u> only.*</li></ul>

* Refer to <u>The Elements of Health: Exercise</u>.

Parasympa (DR) may be needed at any stage of the GAS, as <u>High Autonomic</u> (Sympathetic Dominance) is an underlying cause in most cases.

Take 25 mg of Zinc (more if appropriate based on the <u>Zinc Taste Test</u>) three times a day to lower cortisol levels.

DMAE-H3 is made by TwinLab (available from health food stores). It protects your brain from the harmful effects of excessive cortisol and helps restore memory, concentration, and wellbeing. It sounds like some exotic drug, but is actually a naturally occurring nutrient (primarily from fish). It also balances the autonomic nervous system.

Phosphatidylserine can be a critical nutrient to restoring adrenal function. It is expensive and I will usually skip using it unless adrenal function doesn't improve after using other approaches. It is, however, remarkably effective for lowering cortisol levels and restoring normal cortisol rhythm. It also improves concentration, short-term memory, energy and mood, restores dopamine levels (a neurotransmitter normally depleted by chronic stress), protects the myelin sheath around nerves, balances the autonomic nervous system, and increases the nerve growth factor for repair of nerves damaged by excess cortisol.

If cost isn't an issue or you've already done everything else and aren't improving, definitely include phosphatidylserine. Take 2-4 capsules twice a day.

DHEA is not recommended unless you have labwork indicating you need it. Using the programs outlined on the preceding page, you should see a measurable improvement in your health within six weeks, as evidenced by follow-up Health Graphs, Home Tests, and Lab Tests.

Don't take progesterone cream for more than three months without getting tested for your progesterone levels. (See Using Lab Tests: Specialty Tests To Consider.) Excessive supplementation of progesterone cream can upset male and female hormone levels and predispose to depression.

Be patient; Adrenal Dysfunction usually takes many years to develop. Give your body time to heal. Within two to six weeks you should know if you're on the right track.

I recommend making use of the Health Graph and Home Tests every four to six weeks. Retest more frequently, if you prefer. Your lab work should be re-checked every three to six months until it's balanced, then every six to twelve months after that.

Restoring adrenal function can be a very complicated process because there is so much involved. Despite having very powerful and very consistently effective tools in your hands through this workbook, you may need the guidance of a physician to find the answer to the puzzle.

If you're not seeing any results after six weeks, get an adrenal function test to measure cortisol levels, cortisol rhythm, DHEA, and DHEA/Cortisol ratio. (See Using Lab Tests: Specialty Test Info.) The results will often indicate what needs to be done. I run adrenal function tests on my patients whenever the findings from office exams aren't clear, or when there has been no improvement after the six-week trial period.

When you order an adrenal function test from *The Elements of Health*, I will analyze the interpretation and give you a written report with recommendations. Often this report will offer the answers you've been seeking.

Balancing very complex adrenal problems is outside the scope of this workbook. If you find you're not making progress, consider seeing a physician trained in the Functional Medicine approach.

Y̶ou can solve vitamin and mineral deficiencies by being disciplined about the food you eat. When using foods to balance your nutrition, you are getting vitamins and minerals in their most natural, most available, and most effective form.

A customized, nutrient-rich diet will allow you to decrease your use of supplements as your health improves. Your ultimate goal is to have your diet meet most of your nutritional needs. This way, you will be training yourself to eat in ways that support your overall health and meet your specific needs.

As you go through the following lists, note the sources of vitamins and minerals are in whole, natural foods. Pizza, soda, hamburgers, hot dogs, pastries, cookies, candies, and a long list of other refined foods are not on the list. These foods are what I call entertainment — fun, but not at all nutritious. It's okay to eat them once in a while (at least I hope so, because I do). Just remember, you can't be truly healthy living on refined foods. Most of your diet should consist of whole foods in their natural state.

Vitamins: Functions and Food Sources

Vitamin	Functions	Deficiency Symptoms	Sources
A	Resistance to infection, protects mucous membranes (digestive tract, lungs, etc.), vision, secretion of enzymes and hormones, antioxidant.	Frequent infections, inflammation of lungs and intestines, poor teeth and gums, skin and hair problems, fatigue.	Fruits and vegetables, fertile eggs, butter, whole milk, fish liver oils.
B1 — Thiamine	Protein metabolism, nervous system, producing energy in the cells, improves energy and stamina, protects the heart.	Loss of appetite, muscle weakness, fatigue, irritability, slow heartbeat, low blood pressure, diabetes, soreness, depression, weak digestion.	Nutritional yeast, wheat germ, whole grains, nuts and seeds (and their butters), beans, milk and milk products.
B2 — Riboflavin	Normal growth and repair of cells; health of eyes, skin, hair, and nails.	Bloodshot eyes, itching and burning of eyes, sore tongue, inflammation of skin or mucous membranes, cracked lips.	Milk, nutritional yeast, cheese, whole grains, nuts and seeds, wheat germ.
B3 — Niacin	Circulation, nervous system, protein and carbohydrate metabolism, dilates blood vessels and increases the flow of blood (especially hands and feet).	Nervousness, irritability, insomnia, poor memory, depression, cold hands and feet, forgetfulness, headaches, digestive problems, diarrhea.	Nutritional yeast, wheat germ, nuts and seeds, green vegetables, whole brown rice, liver.

Vitamins: Functions and Food Sources (continued)

Vitamin	Functions	Deficiency Symptoms	Sources
B5 — Pantothenic Acid	Adrenal gland function, nerve function, and manufacture of acetylcholine.	Chronic fatigue, tendency to infections, depression, low blood sugar, allergies, asthma.	Nutritional yeast, wheat germ, whole grains, liver, egg yolk, beans, green vegetables.
B6 — Pyridoxine	Protein and essential fatty acid metabolism, nerve function, action of enzymes, synergist to B12, magnesium, zinc; blood sugar, and cholesterol.	Edema, depression, nervousness, insomnia, headaches, fatigue, irritability, kidney stones, eczema, anxiety.	Wheat germ, nutritional yeast, milk, egg yolks, liver, blackstrap molasses, green leafy vegetables, walnuts, bananas. Cooking and food processing destroys B6.
B12 — Cobalamin	Production of red blood cells, growth in kids, health of nervous system, production and function of enzymes.	Pernicious anemia, chronic fatigue, numbness and stiffness, poor concentration, lack of appetite, and poor growth.	Milk, eggs, meat, kelp, sunflower seeds, blue green algae, spirulina.
B13 — Orotic Acid	Manufacture of nucleic acids, regeneration of cells.	Premature aging, degenerative illnesses of various kinds.	Whey portion of milk; more available when the milk is soured (cultured).
B15 — Pangamic Acid	Increases oxygen uptake of cells, increases fat metabolism, regulates nervous system, energy production in cells, tonifies glands.	Heart disease, fatigue, lack of libido, high cholesterol, muscle cramping, nerve dysfunction, poor circulation, premature aging.	Nuts and seeds, brown rice, whole grains.
Bio-flavonoids	Strengthens capillaries, anticoagulant, synergist to Vitamin C, balances hormones, immune response.	Easily bruised, frequent and prolonged infections, varicose veins, hemorrhoids, bleeding gums, skin problems, vascular headaches, retinal hemorrhage.	Fresh, raw fruits and vegetables especially the pith (white part) of citrus, bell peppers, cayenne pepper, apricots, strawberries, cherries, grapes.
Biotin	Metabolism of proteins and fats, health of hair	Anemia, poor appetite, eczema, hair loss, dandruff, fatigue, depression.	Normally produced in the intestinal tract if healthy flora is present nutritional yeast, brown rice, soybeans, organ meats.

Vitamins: Functions and Food Sources *(continued)*

Vitamin	Functions	Deficiency Symptoms	Sources
C	Formation of connective tissues (collagen), antioxidant, gland function (especially adrenals and thyroid), detixifies toxins, immune system; healthy teeth, bones, and gums.	Joint and muscle problems, frequent prolonged infections, bad teeth and gums, anemia, slow wound healing, easily bruised, low adrenals and thyroid.	Fresh fruits and vegetables, especially citrus, apples, strawberries, bell peppers, cherries, tomatoes, broccoli, guava, potatoes, and cabbage.
Choline	Component of lecithin, fat metabolism (including fat-soluble vitamins), production of proteins, nerve function.	High cholesterol, arteriosclerosis, liver and gall bladder dysfunction, poor nerve function.	Lecithin, wheat germ, nutritional yeast, egg yolks, beans, dark leafy greens.
D	Absorption of calcium and phosphorus, parathyroid gland function, formation and maintenance of teeth and bones.	Osteoporosis, tooth decay, gum disease, fatigue, muscle weakness, lack of growth in kids.	Fish-liver oils (cod liver oil), milk, butter, egg yolks, seeds (and their sprouts), sunshine.
E	Oxygenates tissues; protects essential fatty acids, antioxidant, protects male and female hormones and fat-soluble vitamins, dilates blood vessels, regulates blood-clotting (thins the blood), glycogen storage in muscles.	Heart disease, lung disease, strokes, infertility, lack of libido, miscarriage, muscle disorders, phlebitis, asthma, fatigue, lack of endurance.	Natural, cold-pressed oils (especially wheat germ oil), whole grains, nuts, and seeds, eggs, green leafy vegetables.
F or Essential Fatty Acids	Regulates immune system, controls inflammation, balances blood clotting, regulates hormones, increases rate of metabolism, delivers calcium to the cells, contributes to health of cell membranes and skin.	Prostate and menstrual disorders, acne, eczema, dry skin, hair, psoriasis, low metabolism, high cholesterol, fatigue, frequent and prolonged infections, heart attacks and strokes, joint and muscle pain.	Cold pressed oils, especially from flax, sesame, wheat germ, walnut, olive, and fish-liver oils (cod and salmon liver oils), butter, egg yolks, nuts, and seeds.
Folic Acid	Synergist to B12, cell division and growth, general metabolism and growth, prevents arteriosclerosis, maintenance of skin and hair.	Intestinal disorders, menstrual problems, premature graying of hair, frequent infections.	Green leafy vegetables, nutritional yeast, wheat germ, nuts, mushrooms, broccoli.
Inositol	Hair, component of lecithin (controls fat metabolism), heart muscle, nerve function.	Eczema, hair loss, high cholesterol, obesity, insulin resistance, constipation.	Lecithin, nutritional yeast, wheat germ, milk, nuts, whole grains (oats), blackstrap molasses.

Vitamins: Functions and Food Sources *(continued)*

Vitamin	Functions	Deficiency Symptoms	Sources
K	Aids liver function, production of prothrombin (blood clotting), and energy production in the tissues	Fatigue, abnormal bleeding (nosebleeds, ulcerative colitis, or stomach ulcers with bleeding), bruise too easily.	Manufactured by healthy gut flora; dark leafy green vegetables, egg yolks, milk, alfalfa, kelp.
PABA	Cell metabolism, healthy skin and hair.	Anemia, eczema, vitiligo, unhealthy skin and hair, fatigue.	Nutritional yeast, whole grains, milk, eggs, wheat germ, molasses.
T	Manufacture of blood platelets, immune function, memory.	Poor immunity, fatigue, hemophilia, anemia.	Sesame seeds and butter (tahini), egg yolks, butter.
U	Protects the health of lining of the intestines.	Stomach ulcers, ulcerative colitis, Crohn's disease (inflammation of intestines).	Cabbage, cabbage juice, sauerkraut, cole slaw.

Minerals: Functions and Food Sources

Mineral	Functions	Deficiency Symptoms	Sources
Calcium (Ca)	An electrolyte that contributes to muscle activity, bones and teeth, growth, and metabolism in cells.	Osteoporosis, nervousness, insomnia, depression, muscle spasms, irritability.	Milk and milk products, dark leafy green vegetables, sesame seeds, oats, almonds.
Chloride (Cl)	An electrolyte that contributes to cell membrane transport, nerve function, and production of digestive enzymes.	Poor digestion, edema, fatigue.	Natural sea salt, tomatoes, celery, cucumber, oats, pineapple, cabbage.
Chromium (Cr)	Works with insulin to control blood sugar, controls cholesterol, a part of enzymes and hormones.	Diabetes, insulin resistance, hypoglycemia, obesity, heart disease, fatigue, arteriosclerosis, male and female. hormone imbalances.	Nutritional yeast, whole grains (wheat germ), mushrooms, raw sugar cane juice (Succanat®).

Minerals: Functions and Food Sources *(continued)*

Mineral	Functions	Deficiency Symptoms	Sources
Copper (Cu)	A synergist with iron, contributes to the production of proteins and connective tissue, health of nerves, thyroid.	Anemia, fatigue, lack of endurance, underactive thyroid, loss of hair, graying of hair.	Green leafy vegetables, whole grains, raisins, liver, beans, almonds.
Iodine (I)	Production of thyroid and female hormones.	Goiter, fatigue, low blood pressure, obesity, frequent and prolonged infections, problems at change of seasons, skin cracks on the hands or feet, excess or thick mucous secretions, sinus infections, skin problems (especially thickening of skin), ovarian dysfunction, benign breast cysts and fibroids, acne, and boils.	Sea vegetables (kelp, nori, dulse, akame, etc.), natural sea salt, seafood, fish-liver oils, egg yolks, garlic.
Iron (Fe)	Production of hemoglobin (carries oxygen in blood).	Anemia, fatigue, no endurance, cold hands and feet, blue tint to the whites of the eyes, headaches, pale skin.	Egg yolks, spinach, alfalfa, beets, nuts and seeds, whole grains.
Magnesium (Mg)	An electrolyte which contributes to the manufacture and action of enzymes, manufacture of proteins, and utilization of essential fatty acids.	Muscle cramping, heart disease, depression, inflammation (arthritis, allergies, asthma, etc.), anxiety, and irritability.	Dark green leafy vegetables, alfalfa, figs, nuts, and seeds (especially sesame seeds and almonds), whole grains.
Lithium (Li)	Regulation of nervous system ("firing threshold" of nerves), hormone receptor regulation, immune function, may prevent atherosclerosis; accumulates in pituitary, thyroid, adrenals, and ovaries, production of nitric oxide.	Depression, manic depression (bipolar disorder, anxiety, fibromyalgia, gout, high or low adrenal, insulin resistance, high thyroid, dysinsulinism, male and female hormonal imbalances, high blood pressure, infertility, chronic viral infections, impotence.	Nutritional yeast, hard water (especially from glacial runoff), whole grains (especially from grains grown in Deaf Smith County, Texas), seafoods, beef liver.

Minerals: Functions and Food Sources *(continued)*

Mineral	Functions	Deficiency Symptoms	Sources
Manganese (Mn)	Production of energy from carbohydrates, makes fats available for burning as energy, maintains strong connective tissues, nerve function, pituitary, thyroid, ovary, testes, and immune function.	Digestive problems, hormone imbalances, fatigue, overweight, infertility, menstrual disorders, low libido, weak ligaments and joints, cyclic fever, virus, goiter, poor resistance to infection, carbohydrate sensitivity, diabetes.	Dark green leafy vegetables, apricots, blueberries, citrus, whole grains, wheat germ, kelp, peas, egg yolks.
Phosphorus (P)	Calcium solubility and availability, balances pH and blood clotting, nerve function, producing energy.	Soft bones and teeth, fatigue, stiffness and achiness (especially thick blood, poor memory, lack of libido.	Whole grains, beans, nutritional yeast, nuts and seeds, egg yolks, milk and milk products.
Potassium (K)	An electrolyte which maintains the acid-alkaline balance in the body, muscle contraction, nerve function, and cell membrane transport.	Nervousness and anxiety, shortness of breath, heart rate too fast (tachycardia), muscle spasm (including heart), cardiovascular dysfunction, high blood pressure, constipation, edema, fatigue.	Fruits and vegetables, milk, nuts, and seeds.
Rubidium (Rb)	May be involved in enzyme reactions.	Cognitive problems (especially in older folks), chronic fatigue, low thyroid.	Vegetables, whole grains, beans.
Selenium (Se)	Synergist with vitamin E and sulfur as an antioxidant.	Poor resistance to infection, inflammatory conditions (arthritis, colitis, bursitis, allergies) Low Thyroid, heart disease	Nutritional yeast, garlic, kelp and sea vegetables, milk and milk products, eggs, mushrooms, whole grains.
Sodium (Na)	An electrolyte which contributes to cell membrane transport, nerve function, glandular function, and production of digestive enzymes	Exhaustion (especially after exposure to heat), nausea, inability to concentrate (thyroid, adrenals, ovaries, testes) digestive problems, under-active gland function.	Natural sea salt, celery, watermelon, kelp.

Minerals: Functions and Food Sources *(continued)*

Mineral	Functions	Deficiency Symptoms	Sources
Sulfur (S)	Maintenance of skin, hair, and nails, balances enzyme reactions in body, critical for antioxidant action and production of collagen.	Weak and lackluster hair, premature aging of skin, skin problems like acne and eczema, inflammation, weak and brittle nails.	Garlic, onions, radish, mustard, ginger, fish, egg yolks, Celtic salt.
Zinc (Zn)	Cell division and production of proteins, enzymes, and hormones, production of insulin, immune function.	Poor growth, prostate problems, low female and male hormones, depression, loss of senses of taste and smell, white spots in nails, low resistance to colds and infections.	Meat, nutritional yeast, wheat germ, oysters, milk, egg yolks, nuts, and seeds (especially pumpkin seeds).

Y ou don't need nutrient supplements if:

- You eat only whole, fresh-picked foods, organically grown in mineral-rich soils.
- You eat only freshly made foods.
- You get plenty of rest and exercise.
- You're not under excessive emotional stress.
- You breathe fresh air and aren't exposed to toxic chemicals in your environment.
- You have no genetic weaknesses that result in limited digestion and absorption of nutrients from foods.
- You have no problems with absorption and have a perfect balance of healthy intestinal flora.

If you meet all of the above requirements, you don't need any nutrient supplements in your diet.

If you're one of the people who doesn't meet all of the above requirements, you should read on.

Diet supplements can be split into two categories:

- Crystalline-pure — manufactured and isolated nutrients
- Food concentrates — derived from naturally occurring, nutrient-rich foods; also includes co-factor nutrients normally found in the same foods as the primary nutrient

The food-concentrate, food form, and food source supplements are vastly superior over the crystalline-pure forms in most cases because:

- Food-based supplements contain nutrients in the form normally found in food.
- Food-based supplements act in your body like food, whereas crystalline-pure nutrients can have an effect like a drug.
- Food-based nutrients tend to work more efficiently and completely, since all of the naturally occurring synergists are present.
- Food-based nutrients tend to support body function as a whole rather than creating a narrow and specific — and potentially imbalanced — result.
- Food-based nutrients tend to have a more gentle and balanced action in your body, whereas crystalline-pure forms tend to create imbalances in other body functions and deplete synergistic nutrients.

I wrestled with whether or not to recommend specific nutritional supplement products in this workbook. The other option was to make generic recommendations and let you purchase the nutrient from a health food store, grocery store, or pharmacy. Experience proves to me, however, that a great percentage of these nutritional supplements don't deliver the consistent clinical results I expect. It is extremely common that I find patients deficient in the very nutrients they are taking as supplements. In this workbook, you get the very same recommendations I make for my patients.

Having said that, you are welcome to experiment with any nutritional supplement, herb, etc. you feel may be useful. Just be sure to measure its results with the tools you've acquired in this workbook. That way you'll know if it's worth using. Ultimately, the effectiveness of a supplement is all conjecture until it produces results.

There are some great lines from the health food stores. I often recommend products from TwinLab, Spectrum, Enzymatic Therapy, and KAL. Gaia and HerbFarm are excellent herb lines. Outside of the scope of this workbook is information you can obtain from health food stores. Talk with the people there; many have a remarkably good background and can be a great resource. You know enough now to spot the folks who don't know what they're talking about.

Biotics Research Corporation (BRC)

Biotics Research is the one professional-quality supplement company that I've ended up using more than any other, because I'm extremely impressed with the sources they use, the quality of concentrating and formulating, and the thought that's put into the formulas.

Biotics is a primary manufacturer (many companies just bottle and label supplements) and their quality-control is the best I've seen. Biotics is one of the few companies that actually has NDC numbers (National Drug Control numbers) on their labels, because the government recognizes the quality. The amount of each nutrient in the bottle is always more than what is listed on the label; so even if you go past the expiration date, you'll still most likely get what's on the label. Besides, the stuff really works!

Here are some of the other reasons why I use Biotics Research Products:

- All Biotics products are manufactured to pharmaceutical standards of purity (even though Biotics doesn't produce drugs, they are licensed to do so because of their high manufacturing standards).

- Biotics history includes operating a Center for Disease Control (CDC)-licensed genetics and toxicology testing lab. The sophistication of their lab allows Biotics to assure that all of their glandular products (made from animals) are uncontaminated and disease-free.

- Biotics has developed and introduced a number of supplements (SOD and catalase (antioxidant enzymes), octacosanol, vegetable-based Vitamin B15, yeast-free selenium and chromium, emulsified Coenzyme Q10, neonatal glandular preparations, gamma oryzanol- and trans-ferulic acid (FRAC)).

- Biotics has a full-time, on-site research department.

- Vegetable cultures are used in tableting, so that there is complete absorption.

- Fat-soluble nutrients are emulsified for greater absorption.

- Biotics was the first (and is still one of the few) to offer the trace minerals germanium, lithium, vanadium, rubidium, and molybdenum.

Biotics Research Products

All of the Biotics Research (BRC) products I recommend are available from DSD International, 800-232-3183 or 602-944-0104, or directly from doctors endorsing and incorporating the *choosing* HEALTH system with their patients.

ADHS — This product contains vitamins, minerals, and herbs known to support normal adrenal function. ADHS often decreases cortisol, increases DHEA levels, and normalizes your immune function (as measured by Secretory IgA levels). Consider ADHS with high adrenal and insulin resistance. Suggest 1-2 tablets, BID with breakfast and lunch. Pregnant or lactating women should not use this product.

ADP — A standardized extract of oregano, emulsified in a sustained release form. Useful in toxic bowel syndrome, parasites, Candida, and other fungal/yeast problems of the bowel and genital-urinary tract. Also useful for upper-respiratory bacterial or viral infections. 5 tablets, 3 times a day just before meals for one week, then 3 tablets, TID just before meals for four weeks. After 14 days on ADP, add **Biodophilus-FOS** and **Colon Plus Capsules**. For a sore throat, crush two tablets and place in a glass of pure water with 2 drops of **Bio-D Mulsion** and gargle once or twice per day. For parasites, use ADP with **Bromelain Plus CLA**. *Pregnant or lactating women should not use ADP.*

AMINO SPORT — An amino acid formulation designed to create an anabolic state. Useful for bodybuilding and rehabilitation. Product can also be used as a broad-spectrum amino acid formula. 1-4 capsules, TID just before meals.

AQUA MAG-CL — Each teaspoon provides 200 mg of magnesium chloride. Consider using for hypertension (high blood pressure), leg cramps, fatigue, adult-onset diabetes, fibromyalgia, chronic fatigue syndrome, cardiac arrhythmias/tachycardia, emotional stress, anxiety, depression, and panic attacks. 1-3 tsp a day

ARGIZYME — Enzymatically processed organic beet and tillandsia (Silver Spanish Moss) and rice bran in a base of vitamins, minerals, amino acids, molasses and a specially grown biologically active vegetable culture containing trace elements, SOD, and catalase. This product contains the enzyme of **arginase**. Use with benign prostate hypertrophy, hypertension, symptoms of kidney or bladder dysfunction, edema, and male impotency (increases tissue nitrous oxide levels). 2 capsules, TID with meals.

B6 PHOSPHATE — A biologically active form of Vitamin B-6 (16 mg per tablet) in a vegetable culture base. Use with carpal tunnel syndrome, joint pain, trigger finger (use with raw pecans), homocysteinuria, sensitivity to bright light, burning or tingling in the extremities, inability to recall dreams, low SGOT, and/or SGPT and sensitivity to MSG. Vitamin B-6 is a synergist with magnesium and zinc. 1-2 tablets, TID with meals.

B-12 2000 LOZENGES — Contains 2000 micrograms per lozenge, with 800 micrograms of folic acid and 5 mg of phosphorylated B6. Use with anemia, chronic fatigue, homocysteinuria, digestive inflammation, low serum uric acid, elevated MCV or MCH, chronic debilitating problems, diabetes, neuromuscular disorders. 1-3 lozenges per day between meals.

B-12 2000 LOZENGES — Contains 2000 micrograms per lozenge, with 800 micrograms of folic acid and 5 mg of phosphorylated B6. Use with anemia, chronic fatigue, homocysteinuria, digestive inflammation, low serum uric acid, elevated MCV or MCH, chronic debilitating problems, diabetes, neuromuscular disorders. 1-3 lozenges per day between meals.

B-12/FOLATE PLUS — A source of tillandsia (Silver Spanish Moss). Use as a tonic to assist in the conversion of iron to hemoglobin (trace element content), to help normalize hormonal production, and to increase short-term memory in the elderly. 1-2 capsules, TID.

BASIC NINE — A trace element formula containing trace elements obtained from vegetable culture and raw sugar-cane shoots. Contains chromium, rubidium, lithium, molybdenum, selenium, vanadium, silicon, SOD, and catalase. Use with long-term debilitating conditions, glandular hyper- and hypo-function, with malabsorption, distilled water, and where one or more of the trace elements is found to be insufficient in a hair mineral analysis. 1-2 tablets, TID before meals.

BETAINE PLUS HP — A source of high-potency hydrochloric acid and pepsin in a capsule form (700 mg of HCL and 10 mg of pepsin per capsule). For people who need an increased amount of HCL (chronic hypochlorhydria, achlorhydria). 1-2 capsules with each meal.

BETA-PLUS — A source of organic whole beet concentrate and purified bile salts. Use with constipation, biliary insufficiency (light-colored stools) or where the gall bladder has been removed and the symptoms of gall bladder dysfunction are still present (pain over the eyes, pain in the webbing between the right thumb and forefinger, pain between the shoulder blades, gas, bloating, inability to tolerate fats or fried foods, etc.). Cycle the dosage: 1 tablet per meal on day one, 2 tablets per meal on day two, 3 tablets per meal on day three; repeat.

BETA-TCP — This product is the same as **Beta-Plus** except that it does not contain bile salts, but does contain vitamin C from beet source, taurine, and pancrealipase (all known to assist with cholesterol-to-bile acid conversion). Use with biliary stasis where there is no constipation or light-colored stools and the gall bladder has not been removed. Subjective indications for use include pain over the eyes, pain in the webbing between the right thumb and forefinger, pain between the shoulder blades, gas, bloating, inability to tolerate fats or fried foods, or a history of gall bladder attacks where stones were detected or suspected. 2-3 tablets, TID with meals. If gallstones are suspected, consult a physician.

BIO-6 PLUS UNCOATED — Use with pancreatic dysfunction, hyperglycemia, diabetes, or intestinal problems (such as mucous or undigested food in stool). Product is supplied in both the enteric-coated and uncoated forms. Use the uncoated form if the site of action is the proximal small intestine. Use the coated form if the site of action is the medial or distal small intestine. 3 tablets, TID just before meals.

BIO-AE MULSION — 2,000 I.U. of vitamin A per drop (a small amount of vitamin E is added to prevent oxidation) in an emulsified form to increase assimilation and lymphatic absorption. Use with any condition involving free-radical attack, kidney or bladder dysfunction, night blindness, or skin disorders. 2 d in a glass of pure water, TID just before meals. Women who are pregnant or may become pregnant should restrict their total supplementation of Vitamin A to no more than 12,000 IU total intake per day.

BIO-AE MULSION FORTE — This product is identical to **Bio-AE Mulsion** except that it contains 12,500 I.U. of Vitamin A per drop rather than 2,000 I.U. per drop. Use with kidney or bladder problems, night blindness, skin disorders, immune problems (virus, colds, environmental allergy, flu, or bacterial infection), acne, ringing in the ears, and as an antioxidant. At the onset of a cold or flu, use 6 d in a glass of pure water, BID along with Bio-Immunozyme Forte at 2 tablets, 3 times a day with meals and **Bio-C Plus 1000** at 1 tablet every two hours for 48 hours (reduce if diarrhea occurs). After both low and high blood pressure have been ruled out as the cause of ringing in the ears, rule out entrapment of one of the cranial nerves and use Bio-AE Mulsion Forte at 6 drops in a glass of pure water, BID along with Bio-Immunozyme Forte at 1 tablet, TID with meals. Use 6 d, BID for one week, then reduce to 3 d, BID for another week, and then reduce again to 1 d, BID until the problem abates. Continue the Bio-Immunozyme Forte at 1 tablet, TID with meals until the problem abates. Women who are pregnant or may become pregnant should restrict their total daily Vitamin A supplementation to no more than 12,000 IU.

BIO-ANABOLIC PAK — General support for athletes and people involved in rigorous activity. Bodybuilders should add **Amino Sport** at 1 capsule, TID with meals, **Gammanol Forte with FRAC** at 2 tablets, TID and **Multi-Mins** at 1 tablet, TID with meals.

BIO-B 100 — A multiple-B vitamin containing the natural (phosphorylated) forms of B-1, B-2 and B-6. Combines the **B and G factors**. Use with sensitivity to light, sound, smell, chronic need for hydrochloric acid for digestion, night sweats, burning feet, redness of hands or eyes, cracks in the corner of the mouth, red or swollen tongue, blood sugar problems, general lack of energy. Bio-B 100 is a synergist to magnesium and zinc. Use up to 6 tablets, QID.

BIO-3B-G — A multiple B vitamin containing the natural (phosphorylated) forms of B-1, B-2 and B-6. This product is the same as **Bio-B 100**, except that it is three times higher in natural thiamine (B1). Consider **Bio-3B-G** at 2 tablets, TID where increased thiamine is required (low blood pressure, psychological stress, hypoglycemia, Low Adrenal, and severe fatigue).

BIO-CLA — Each capsule contains 600 mg of Conjugated Linoleum Acid (CLA) extracted from high-linoleic acid containing sunflower and safflower oil. Developed by scientists at the University of Wisconsin's Food Research Institute, CLA has been shown to improve cell metabolism by helping the body reduce fat levels and increase muscle retention. 1-2 capsules, TID before meals.

BIO-C PLUS 1000 — Contains mixed acerbates and citrus lemon bioflavinoids. Product is the same as **Bio-C Plus**, except that each tablet contains 1000 mg of mixed ascorbates rather than 500 mg of mixed ascorbates. 1-2 tablets, TID.

BIO-CARDIOZYME FORTE — A broad-spectrum product designed to support cardio-vascular function. Contains vegetable-culture minerals, phosphorylated forms of B-vitamins and other accessory nutrients known to support cardiac function. Use with cardiac fatigue, muscle weakness, elevated blood pressure, muscle atrophy, and as long-term preventive support. 2-3 tablets, TID with meals. *For severe cardiac stress, add CoQ-Zyme 30 and L-Carnitine Capsules and be under the care of a physician.*

BIOCTASOL FORTE — Each tablet contains 6000 micrograms of octacosanol from a rice source. Allows increased oxygen utilization by muscle and nerve tissue. Use with neuro-muscular degeneration and patients who fail to maintain their manipulative treatments. Product should also be considered for females who desire to become pregnant and have a history of spontaneous abortion. 6 tablets daily.

BIO-CMP — A combination of calcium, magnesium, and potassium. Excellent for muscle and menstrual cramps. Also useful for high adrenal, bursitis, edema, tendonitis, food/environmental sensitivity, exposure to radiation, low-salt diets, and inflammation. 1-2 tablets, TID. With acute muscle or menstrual cramps, use 4 tablets when the cramps begin and then 3 tablets per hour for up to 6 hours.

BIO-CYANIDINS — Contains polyphenols extracted from European pine (Pinus maritima) and grape seed. Consider with ocular degeneration, venous inflammation, capillary fragility, gastric inflammation, increased blood viscosity, and other conditions where a source of polyphenols is required. 1-2 tabs BID

BIODOPHILUS-FOS — Lactobacillus acidophilus (DDS-1) and Bifidobacterium bifidum (3 billion per one-half teaspoon) in a base of fructooligosaccharides (beet source). Use with any condition requiring re-establishment of correct bowel flora (parasites, fungal/yeast overgrowth, gastric inflammation, anti-biotic therapy, constipation, diarrhea). 2-4 capsules just before meals, or ½ to 1 teaspoon, once or twice daily just before meals. With fungal/yeast problems, use only after the patient has been on **ADP** and/or **F/C Cidal** for two weeks.

BIO-D MULSION — Natural Vitamin D in an emulsified liquid form. Synergistic with calcium and magnesium. Use with diastolic hypotension, parathyroid dysfunction, bone healing, osteoporosis, patients who avoid the sun or are housebound, fibroids, and endometriosis. 1-2 d in a glass of pure water, BID or TID with meals. This product is also effective in some cases of psoriasis when applied topically.

BIO-E MULSION FORTE — Natural Vitamin E in a low-dose emulsified liquid form (6 I.U. per drop). Use with muscle and ligament weakness, chronic viral or bacterial problems, cardiac stress, angina, and topically for skin lesions to help prevent scarring (acne, burns, abrasions). 2-3 d in a glass of pure water, BID or TID just before meals.

BIO-FCTS — Each capsule contains 400 mg of sprouted buckwheat culture, 75 mg of Vitamin C (beet source), 100 mg of Quercitin, 10 mg of citrus bioflavinoids, 25 mg of green tea extract, 10 mg of neonatal thymus, and 5 mg of neonatal spleen in a base of Oorganik-15, SOD, and catalase. Use with virus (to prevent reverse transcription), diabetes (to block the sorbitol pathway), capillary fragility, tinnitus, vascular headaches, hemorrhoids, and macular degeneration. 2 capsules, BID.

BIO-GGG-B — Contains 300 percent of the R.D.A. of the "G" factors (riboflavin) and 100 percent of the R.D.A. of the "B" factors (thiamine) in a phosphorylated form, along with other components of B complex. Consider this product when the need for increased levels of riboflavin is present (night sweats, redness of the palms or soles of the feet, edema, digestive inflammation, hypertension, muscle spasms, and non-toxic goiter). 2-4 tablets, TID just before meals.

BIO-GLYCOZYME FORTE — A broad-spectrum product designed to support reactive hypoglycemia, adrenal fatigue, general fatigue, stress, highly refined diets, and carbohydrate sensitivity. Contains phosphorylated forms of B-1, B-2 and B-6, neonatal bovine glandular and organ components, chromium, vanadium, zinc, magnesium, and other accessory nutrients. 2-3 tablets, TID at 10:00 a.m., 3:00 p.m. and 2 hours after supper. If the patient is able to fall asleep but cannot remain asleep, add 3 tablets just before bedtime.

BIO-HPF (H-pylori formula) — A broad-spectrum herbal-based formula designed to ameliorate gastric inflammation and erosion caused by H-pylori bacteria. Recent (1999) clinical studies have shown the product to be effective (by reducing or eliminating the antigen) in over 80 percent of the cases where H-pylori has been identified (by serum and stool testing). 2 capsules, TID just before meals. Should be considered with **Gastrazyme** and **ADP**.

BIO-IMMUNOZYME FORTE — A broad-spectrum product containing vitamins, minerals, enzymes, as well as neonatal bovine glandular and organ components known to support immune function. Product is in a base of SOD, catalase, echinacea, methyl donors, and chlorophyll. In the acute phase, use 2-3 tablets, TID or QID with food. In the chronic phase, use 1 tablet, TID with meals. For Hepatitis A, B or C, use with **Cytozyme-THY** — 4 tablets, QID with meals, **Livotrit-Plus** — 2 tablets, TID with meals, **BioProtect** — 1 capsule, TID with meals, **Dismuzyme Plus Granules** — 1 teaspoon, TID with meals, **IAG**, 2-6 tablespoons daily, **Beta-TCP** — 2 tablets, TID with meals and **Cytozyme-LV** — 2 tablets, TID with meals. ***With any severe immune problem, especially hepatitis, you need to be under the care of a physician.***

BIO-MEGA 3 — Each capsule contains 1000 mg of natural marine-lipid concentrate, providing a natural source of 180 mg of eicosapentaenoic acid (EPA) and 120 mg of docosahexaeonic acid (DHA). Consider with increased fibrinogen (tendency to blood clotting), rheumatoid arthritis, systemic inflammation, atherosclerosis, and other autoimmune problems. 1-2 capsules, TID.

BIO-MULTI PLUS — A broad-spectrum multiple vitamin and mineral formula containing emulsified forms of the fat-soluble vitamins, mixed ascorbates, and vegetable culture forms of trace elements. Excellent for long-term preventive support and as a synergist for specific nutritional programs. For long-term application, use 3 tablets a day (two in the morning with a meal and one at night). As a synergist with other nutritional programs or for short-term use where higher-nutrient levels are required, use 2 tablets, TID with meals for 30 days.

BIOPROTECT — A multiple-nutrient formula designed to provide broad-spectrum anti-oxidant support. Unlike the synthetic beta carotene or mixed carotenoids found in other products, BioProtect provides a full-spectrum blend of the natural carotenoids, beta-carotene, alpha carotene, lycopene, zeaxanthin, crytoxanthin, and lutein. Helps prevent free-radical damage from pollution, tobacco smoke, synthetic building materials, electromagnetic radiation, and psychological and physical stress. 1-2 capsules, TID with meals. When higher levels of anti-oxidant protection are required, use with **GSH-Plus**. 1 capsule, TID with meals.

BIO-SOY FLAVONES — Each capsule contains 50 mg of soy flavones (Genistein, Daidzein, and Glycitein) in a vegetable-culture base containing SOD and catalase. Consider with breast cancer or females genetically pre-disposed to estrogen-initiated tumors, menopausal hot flashes, osteoporosis, and general cardiovascular support. 1-2 capsules daily just before meals.

BLACK CURRANT SEED OIL — A source of GLA (40 mg per capsule). Use with inflammation, hypertension due to vasoconstriction, uterus constriction, skin conditions (eczema), muscle cramps, and menstrual cramps. Synergist with zinc, Vitamin B-6, and magnesium. 1-2 capsules, TID with meals. During acute menstrual cramps, use 4 capsules, TID with meals.

BROMELAIN PLUS — A source of lactose-free bromelain. Use for inflammation and infant digestive problems. For infant digestive distress, use 1 crushed tablet, BID with food. For adult inflammation, use 3 tablets, TID on an empty stomach. If the inflammation is acute, increase to 5 tablets, TID on an empty stomach.

BROMELAIN PLUS CLA — Source of lactose-free bromelain. This product is the same as **Bromelain Plus**, except that Bromelain Plus CLA also contains cellulase, lipase, ficin, and amylase. Use with symptoms of intestinal parasites, mucous, pancreatic dysfunction, tissue trauma, or inflammation (a vegetarian alternative to **Intenzyme Forte**). 3 tablets, TID on an empty stomach. If problem is acute, increase to 5 tablets, TID on an empty stomach.

BUTYRIC/CAL-MAG — A source of butyric acid. Use with probiotics (**Lactozyme**, **Colon Plus**, and/or **Biodophilus-FOS**). Increased butyric acid levels are associated with decreased risk to colon cancer. This product has also been used successfully with some cases of chronic fatigue syndrome. 1-2 capsules, TID just before meals.

B-VITAL — Each capsule contains 750 mg of Peruvian Maca root and 50 mg of Elk Antler Velvet (from live American elk.) ***B-Vital*** should be considered as adjunctive supplemental support with lack of libido (male and female), reduced testosterone, menopausal hot flashes, and lack of stamina. ***A research study showed 100% of the men in the study taking B-Vital experienced an increase in testosterone levels.*** 1 capsule, BID.

CA-ZYME — A source of calcium citrate (200 mg per tablet). Use in situations where calcium alone is required (that is, magnesium with the calcium is contraindicated). 3 tablets, TID on an empty stomach.

CA/MG ZYME — A source of calcium citrate and magnesium aspartate in a ratio of 5 parts of calcium to 1 part of magnesium. Use with muscle cramps, for long-term calcium supplementation, fever, increased secretions, autonomic imbalance, high endocrine glands, low blood calcium, skin conditions (itching, lesions), excessive bleeding (menses, nose). 2-3 tablets, TID on an empty stomach. With fever or acute muscle cramps, use 3-6 tablets per hour until the problem abates and then begin to reduce.

CA/MG PLUS — A source of calcium citrate and magnesium aspartate in a ratio of 5 parts of calcium to 1 part of magnesium. This is the same basic formula as **CA/MG Zyme**, except that each tablet contains 1 mg of bovine parathyroid tissue. Use with parathyroid dysfunction, blood-calcium-to-phosphorus ratio weighted to the phosphorus side, joint stiffness, tissue/muscle tenderness, severe muscle cramps, chronic stiff neck, chronic upper-respiratory mucous, chronic digestive dysfunction, and hoarseness. 1-2 tablets, TID just before meals.

CAPRICIN — Each capsule contains a minimum of 400 mg of caprylic acid. Designed to be used alone or in conjunction with **F.C. Cidal** and **ADP** in difficult cases of fungal/yeast overgrowth and as a supplemental source of calcium and magnesium (300 mg of calcium and 150 mg of magnesium per capsule). Unlike ADP and F.C. Cidal, **Capricin** can be used during pregnancy and lactation. 2-3 capsules, TID with meals.

CHONDROPLUS — A source of manganese, purified chondroitin sulfates, and Vitamin B-12 (synergist with manganese). Excellent for ligament, disc and cartilage support, athletic injuries, and long-term preventive support for athletes or people engaged in strenuous activity. 1-2 tablets, TID with meals. Increase to 4 tablets, QID in acute situations.

CHONDROSAMINE PLUS — Three capsules contain 1000 mg of glucosamine as glucosamine HCl.

CHONDROSAMINE-S — Three capsules contain 600 mg of glucosamine from glucosamine sulfate. Both products also contain 500 mg of **Purified Chondroitin Sulfate**, 180 mg of beet-source Vitamin C, 25 mg of silica from raw cane, 6 mg of manganese, 45 mg of pantothenic acid, 50 mg of niacinamide, 100 mg of MSM, 200 mcg of folic acid, 3 mcg of Vitamin B-12 (hydroxycobalamin), 20 mcg of SOD, and 20 mcg of catalase. This product should be considered for osteo- and rheumatoid arthritis, joint inflammation, cartilage repair, and any other condition where increased sulfur intake is needed. 1-2 capsules, TID with meals.

CHLOROCAPS — A source of fat- and water-soluble chlorophyll and Vitamin K. Use for internal healing, inflammation, toxemia, I.C.V. problems, arthritis, and anemia. 1 capsule, TID with meals. Use 1 capsule in an ounce of distilled water as a lavage for sinusitis. *Due to the Vitamin K component, Chlorocaps should not be used if the patient is on blood-thinning medication*.

CHROMIUM, AQUEOUS — Each drop supplies 150 mcg of trivalent chromium in a rapidly absorbed liquid form. Use with both decreased and increased blood sugar levels, morning sickness, low HDL with high cholesterol, pancreatic dysfunction, and general fatigue. 1-2 d per day

CHROMIUM PICOLINATE — Each capsule supplies 200 mcg of chromium picolinate and 2 mg of vitamin B-6. This is a well-absorbed form of chromium for use with bodybuilding, weight-loss programs, decreased and increased blood sugar levels, and morning sickness. 1-2 capsules, 3 times daily.

COLON PLUS CAPSULES AND POWDER — Contains psyllium, flax seed, apple pectin, lactobacillus acidophilus, bromelain, and other nutrients known to help normalize bowel flora and function. Use with constipation, diarrhea, gas, bloating and other non-obstructive bowel problems. 1 tsp in a glass of pure warm water in the morning and evening, or 5 capsules, TID just before meals.

COQ-ZYME FORTE — 10 mg of emulsified Coenzyme Q10 per tablet. Use where increased oxygenation is required, i.e., cardiac stress, immune dysfunction, periodontal disease, high blood pressure, allergies, asthma, multiple sclerosis, diabetes, ulcers, and viral infections. 1-2 tablets, TID with meals.

COQ-ZYME 30 — 30 mg of emulsified Coenzyme Q10. Use where increased oxygenation is required, i.e., cardiac stress, immune dysfunction, periodontal disease, high blood pressure, allergies, asthma, multiple sclerosis, diabetes, ulcers, and viral infections. 1 tablet, TID with meals. *Note:* The emulsified Coenzyme Q10 produced by Biotics Research will raise blood levels an average of three times higher than any of the dry forms.

CR-ZYME — A source of non-yeast chromium from vegetable culture. Contains 200 mcg of the Glucose Tolerance Factor per tablet. Use with morning sickness, decreased and increased blood glucose levels, elevated cholesterol with low HDL, pancreatic dysfunction, and as a co-factor to zinc and vanadium. 1-2 tablets, TID with meals.

CU-ZYME — Copper gluconate and aspartate complexed with protein to aid in the assimilation of the copper. Use with inflammation, amoebic infections, low HDL, copper anemia, or ovarian dysfunction where a known copper insufficiency is present. 1-2 tablets a day with meals. If zinc is also being used supplementally, ensure that the CU-Zyme is given at a different time than the zinc (these two minerals compete for absorption). If copper is to be used for over 60 days, ensure that **FE-Zyme** is used in lieu of CU-Zyme, as it is a balanced zinc, copper, and iron formula.

CYTOZYME-AD — A source of neonatal bovine adrenal. Use with chronic fatigue, hypoglycemia, craving for salt, lowered resistance from long-term illness, flu, colds, hypotension (use with **Bio-Glycozyme Forte** and **Bio-D Mulsion**), asthma, inflammation, allergy/sensitivity to foods or environmental toxins, lack of ligament strength (patient is unable to hold a manipulative treatment), ridges in the fingernails, and patients who are unable to work under pressure or become enraged easily. 1-2 tablets, TID with meals. With severe hypotension, 1 tablet, 8 times a day should be considered.

CYTOZYME-B — A source of neonatal bovine brain with the pineal, pituitary, and hypothalamus intact. Use with brain injury, loss of memory, nightmares, epilepsy, dementia, and mental fatigue from psychological stress. 1-2 tablets, TID with meals. Increase if the problem is acute.

CYTOZYME-F (Female) — A source of raw bovine ovarian tissue combined with other glandular components known to support the female endocrine functions. Use as broad-spectrum support for female glandular function. 1-2 tablets, TID with meals.

CYTOZYME-H — A source of neonatal bovine heart. Use with cardiac stress, fatigue, lack of muscle tone or integrity, or to increase muscle demand for glucose and some cases of fibromyalgia. 1-2 tablets, TID with meals. In some cases of fibromyalgia, up to 20 tablets a day may be required to resolve tissue inflammation and tenderness.

CYTOZYME-KD — A source of neonatal bovine kidney. Use with edema, renal dysfunction, hypertension, severe diastolic hypotension, and toxemia. 1-2 tablets, TID with meals.

CYTOZYME-LV — A source of toxin-free neonatal bovine liver. Use with general liver dysfunction, virus, edema, and as a source of B vitamins. 2-3 tablet, TID with meals.

CYTOZYME-M (Male) — A source of raw bovine orchic tissue, combined with other glandular components known to support male endocrine function. Use for broad-spectrum male endocrine support. 1-2 tablets, TID with meals.

CYTOZYME-O — Raw bovine ovarian tissue. Use with delayed puberty, menses problems (amenorrhea or excessive bleeding), cramps, and hot flashes. 1 tablet, TID with meals.

CYTOZYME-ORCHIC — Raw bovine orchic tissue. Use with orchitis, lack of fertility in men, gynecomastia (breasts on men), testicular atrophy, lack of sex drive, or low sperm count (for low sperm count use with **Bio-Immunozyme Forte**). 1 tablet, TID.

CYTOZYME-PAN — A source of neonatal bovine pancreas. Use with diabetes, wasting diseases, pancreatitis, insulin resistance, ulcers, and dysinsulinism. 1-2 tablets, TID with meals. **With the exception of insulin resistance, you need to be under the care of a physician for any of the above-listed conditions.**

CYTOZYME PAROTID-TS — Contains 200 mg of bovine parotid, 10 mg of neonatal thymus, and 10 mg of spleen. Use for iodine sensitivity, thick saliva, diminished saliva, reduced or abnormal sperm count, non-toxic goiter, food and environmental allergies or sensitivities, exposure to xenobiotics (pesticides, herbicides, plastics, etc.), poor absorption, and some types of digestive problems. 1 tablet, TID

CYTOZYME-PT/HPT — A source of neonatal bovine pituitary and hypothalamus. Use with low or high pituitary, stomach problems, high or low adrenal, insomnia, epilepsy, anorexia, inability to gain or lose weight, low thyroid secondary to low pituitary, insulin resistance, and neuro-muscular disorders. 1-2 tablets, TID with meals.

CYTOZYME-SP — A source of neonatal bovine spleen. Use with free-radical problems, spleen dysfunction, immune insufficiency, increased or decreased red blood values, and increased or decreased serum iron. 1-2 tablets, TID.

CYTOZYME-THY — A source of neonatal bovine thymus. Use with viral or bacterial infections, immune insufficiency, low gamma globulin, sensitivity to milk products, croup, inflammation, high thyroid, wound healing, lymph edema, and myasthenia gravis. 1-2 tablets, TID with meals. Increase to 4 tablets, QID during the acute phase of any infection and with Hepatitis A, B, or C. **For myasthenia gravis or hepatitis, you need to be under the care of a physician.**

CYTOZYME-TRACHEA — Concentrated bovine trachea from neonatal bovine source. Consider Cytozyme-Trachea at 3 capsules, TID and 4 capsules at bedtime (9 grams per day) for arthritic conditions, free-radical pathology (research conducted by John Prudden, MD), and other conditions where shark cartilage would be considered. *Research indicates bovine trachea is as effective as shark cartilage at significantly lower levels (70 grams of shark cartilage daily are required to reach therapeutic levels, versus 9 grams of bovine trachea).*

DE-STRESS — Two capsules supply 220 mg of a bioactive milk-derived peptide, having anxiolytic activity. De-Stress can be used in any case where psychological stress, insomnia, or anxiety are present. 1-2 capsules at bedtime and during the day, as needed for periods of high stress. Human studies indicate De-Stress has no known side-effects and will generally work within 24-48 hours after the initial dose.

DHEA — Each tablet contains 10 mg of DHEA (dehydroepiandosterone). ½-2 tablets daily. *Use where DHEA insufficiency can be demonstrated (saliva, serum, or urine testing) with a decreased cortisol level. Supplemental DHEA should not be used with a decreased DHEA and an increased cortisol. Use the adrenal stress index test to determine whether or not you actually need DHEA. Taking DHEA when you don't need it can be detrimental to your health.*

DISMUZYME PLUS GRANULES — Vegetable-culture source of SOD and catalase. Use with chronic pain, free-radical problems, viral or bacterial infections, rheumatoid arthritis, systemic inflammation, and immune insufficiency. 1-3 tsp daily just before meals.

DL-PHENYLALANINE — 600 mg per capsule. Use with chronic or acute pain and depression. For acute pain, use 1 capsule every two hours. For chronic pain or depression use 2 capsules, 3 times per day with meals.

E-MULSION 200 — 200 mg of emulsified vitamin E per capsule. This product is the same as **Bio-E Mulsion Forte**, except that it contains mixed tocopherols in addition to the d-alpha tocopherol. Use with muscular weakness, muscle cramps occurring upon exertion, ligament weakness, chronic viral or bacterial infections, cardiac stress, to prevent oxidation of LDL cholesterol, benign cysts or fibroids, increased fibrinogen levels, and with intermittent claudication. 1-3 capsules a day.

EQUI-FEM — A source of vitamins, minerals, and glandular components known to support female endocrine functions, in a base of Dong Quai and Black Cohosh. Use with symptoms of PMS, menopausal symptoms, hot flashes, and for general female support. 2 tablets, TID with meals. For hot flashes, use with **B-12/Folate Plus** and **Black Currant Seed Oil**. If the hot flashes are severe, add Liquid Iodine. If the patient is on hormonal replacement therapy, use **PMT** in lieu of **Equi-Fem**. PMT is identical to Equi-Fem, except that it does not contain any organ or glandular components.

F.C. CIDAL — An herbal supplement designed to accompany **ADP** in cases of difficult dysbiosis, yeast/fungal overgrowth, and some types of amoebic parasites. 1-3 capsules, TID just before meals.

FE-ZYME — A source of iron, copper, zinc, and Vitamin B-12 in a base of ascorbic acid to facilitate uptake of the iron. Use with anemia, pregnancy, cold hands and feet due to anemia, blue tint to the whites of the eyes, and as long-term copper, zinc, or iron support (a balanced formula). 1 tablet, 2 or TID with meals.

FLAX SEED OIL — 1000 mg of oil per capsule from certified organically grown, cold-pressed flax seed. Use with increased or decreased blood fats, with immune insufficiency, as a calcium synergist, with prostate hypertrophy, for skin conditions, as cardio-vascular support, with increased fibrinogen levels, and as preventive support where a genetic pre-disposition to free-radical problems is present. 1-2 capsules, TID with meals.

FOLIC ACID 800 — 800 micrograms of folic acid per tablet. Use with anemia, chronic fatigue, digestive inflammation, elevated (gout) or reduced uric acid, elevated MCV or MCH (red blood indices), nerve degeneration, or inflammation. Use as a synergist with Vitamin B-12, Vitamin B-6, zinc, and magnesium. 1 tablet, TID with meals. Increase to 2 tablets, TID with gout. Protectively, folic acid should always be used with Vitamin B-12 (**B-12 2000 Lozenges**).

GAMMANOL FORTE WITH FRAC — A source of gamma oryzanol and free transferulic acid (FRAC). Use with bodybuilding to support lean muscle mass, PMS, menopausal hot flashes, amenorrhea, elevated blood fats, low blood pressure, angina, low adrenal, stomach inflammation, nervous tension, and exposure to free-radical generators such as chemicals and radiation, and where there is a need to increase human growth hormone. 2 tablets, TID with meals. For athletes, use 2-4 tablets before and after a workout and 2 tablets at bedtime. For elevated blood fats, use 4 tablets after each meal. For patients who complain of muscle soreness after sleeping, use 4 tablets at bedtime.

GAMOCTAPRO — A source of high-quality isolated soy protein containing branch-chain amino acids, lecithin, gamma oryzanol, free transferulic acid (FRAC), octacosanol, and bromelain. This product is lactose-free, carbohydrate-free, and for most people is significantly less allergenic than milk or egg-white proteins. An excellent source of protein for patients who are on a reduced-carbohydrate diet (as with insulin resistance), or people who exercise and need a high-quality protein supplement. The combination of nutrients will help increase the food utilization efficiency (more muscle mass gained than with protein alone) and will help support dietary protein breakdown in the digestive system.

GARLIC PLUS — A source of garlic concentrate in a base of Vitamin C and chlorophyll. Use to enhance immune functions, with high blood pressure, for fungal and yeast infections, for prevention of colds and flu, and other viral problems. 1 tablet, TID with meals.

GASTRAZYME — A source of Vitamin U and other nutrients known to oppose inflammation and assist with healing in the gastro-intestinal tract. Use with ulcers, hiatal hernia, acid reflux, excess HCl production, heartburn, sour stomach, and as a source of chlorophyll. 2-3 tablets, TID just before meals. For ulcers, use 6 tablets, TID with meals for 30 days or until the inflammation is resolved and the lesion(s) begin to heal. *With any chronic stomach pain, an ulcer is possible and you need to consult a physician.*

GINKGO BILOBA — A standardized 24% extract of Ginkgo Biloba (40 mg per tablet) containing flavonoid glycosides and ginkgolides, including Ginkgolide B. Use with cerebral vascular insufficiency, i.e., vertigo, poor memory, tinnitus, cloudy thinking, headache, senile dementia, Alzheimer's, macular degeneration, diabetic nerve damage, vascular inflammation, lack of libido, and free-radical problems. 1-2 tablets, TID with meals.

GLUCOBALANCE — A vitamin and mineral combination formulated by Dr. Alan Gaby and Dr. Jonathan Wright. An excellent formula for insulin-dependent diabetics, non-insulin-dependent diabetics, elevated triglycerides with low HDL, and insulin resistance. 2 capsules, TID with meals. *If you are an insulin-dependent diabetic, check your blood sugar levels frequently; Glucobalance often has a dramatic effect on your insulin needs.*

GSH-PLUS — A source of L-glutathione, N-acetylcysteine, and glycine. Use for upper-respiratory inflammation, digestive inflammation, and where increased anti-oxidant protection above that found in **BioProtect** is required. 1 capsule, TID with meals.

GTA — A source of thyroid glandular. Use for low thyroid. Product will perform best if used with **Thyrostim** and **Flax Seed Oil**. 1-2 capsules, TID. If T-3 or T-3 Uptake is decreased, use **GTA** with **Meda-Stim** in lieu of **Thyrostim**. If High Adrenal is present, add **ADHS**.

HCL-PLUS — A source of betaine hydrochloride, glutamic acid, ammonium chloride, pepsin, and Vitamin B-6. Use with a need to acidify systemically (bursitis, tendonitis, and environmental sensitivity (hay fever)), or symptoms of digestive dysfunction (bloating, bad breath, body odor, loss of taste for meat, anemia, pregnancy, or low mineral values as seen on a hair mineral analysis). *Note:* A chronic need for HCl-containing supplements may be an indication of a thiamine (**BIO-3B-G**) or zinc (**ZN-zyme forte**) deficiency. If there is a need to acidify your body, take 1-2 tablets an hour until you notice relief, and then take 2-4 tablets TID.

HYDROZYME — A source of betaine HCl, glutamic acid, ammonium chloride, pepsin, and Vitamin B-6. This product is the same as **HCL-Plus**, except that each tablet also contains 10 mg of pancreatin. Use with chronic indigestion, chronic need for HCl or pancreatic support, bowel dysfunction (diarrhea or constipation), gas, bloating, bad breath, body odor, loss of taste for meat, anemia, pregnancy, and low mineral values as seen in a hair mineral analysis.

IAG — Arabinogalactan derived from the western larch tree. This is an excellent product for chronic immune dysfunction, viruses, inner-ear infections (children), free-radical pathologies, allergy, fibromyalgia, chronic fatigue syndrome, etc. This product should be considered along with **Bio-C Plus 1000** (1-2 tablets daily) and **Liquid Iodine** (10 to 15d daily). Consider 1-2 tsp, TID for chronic problems, and up to 6 teaspoons, TID in the acute phase. For children, consider ½ teaspoon, TID.

IMMUNO-gG — Two capsules contain 240 mg of Immunoglobulin G (from bovine colostrum), 120 mg of lysine, and 60 mg of arginine. This product was formulated to provide immune support for viral conditions, immune compromise in the small intestine (leaky gut), and other immune problems. 2 capsules, TID just before meals. When used with gastric immune problems, this product should be considered with **IAG** and **IPS**.

INOSITOL — Each tablet contains 650 mg of inositol derived from rice. Use with elevated or reduced blood sugar, elevated blood fats, diabetes, skin lesions, slow growth, hair loss that is not genetically pre-determined, pesticide poisoning, lymph edema, and in some cases of constipation. 1 capsule, TID with meals.

INTENZYME FORTE — A source of animal and plant proteolitic enzymes. This product is high in trypsin and chymotrypsin. Use with systemic inflammation, tissue damage, arthritis, food sensitivity, poor circulation due to inflammation, or atherosclerosis (use with **Porphyra-Zyme**), phlebitis, and free-radical conditions. With acute injury, use 10 tablets immediately and then 5 tablets, QID on an empty stomach for 3 days, and then reduce to 4 tablets, TID on an empty stomach until the inflammation and swelling abates. With chronic inflammation, arthritis, etc., use 3-4 tablets, TID on an empty stomach. *Phlebitis is a serious condition and needs to be treated (or at least tracked) by a physician.*

IPS (Intestinal Permeability Support) — An intestinal permeability supplement designed to stimulate growth and repair of the intestinal mucosa as well as aiding in gut detoxification. Each capsule contains glutamine, glucosamine sulfate, Tillandsia root, gamma oryzanol, glutathione, Jerusalem artichoke, lamb intestine concentrate, and vegetable cellulase. Consider using the product with **Nutri-Clear** and **Beta-TCP** or **Beta-Plus**. 2-4 capsules, BID one hour before meals.

IRON AND COPPER FREE MULTI-MINS — A source of organically derived minerals (contains both macro and micro minerals). HCl is added to facilitate breakdown of the minerals. This product is the same as **Multi-Mins**, except that it contains no iron or copper. Use where a broad-spectrum organically-combined multiple-mineral formula with no iron or copper is required. Product contains HCl to assist with absorption of the minerals. 1-2 tablets, TID with meals.

IRON AND COPPER FREE MULTI-PLUS — This product is the same as **Bio-Multi Plus**, except it contains no iron or copper. Use where a broad-spectrum multiple-vitamin, multiple-mineral formula without iron and copper is required. 3 tablets a day; best taken with each meal, but 2 tablets in the morning with a meal and 1 tablet in the evening is okay. *All men over 40 years of age should consider taking multiple-vitamin and -mineral formulas that are iron- and copper-free. This is because men tend to build up iron and copper in their bodies as they get older, and it makes them more likely to have a heart attack or stroke.*

K-ZYME — A source of organically derived potassium and potassium gluconate (99 mg per tablet). Use with sympathetic dominance, frequent sighing, breathlessness, dry mouth, gag easily, tachycardia, high pituitary, thyroid, or adrenal. 1-2 tablets, TID with meals.

LACTOZYME — Each tablet supplies 5 to 6 million freeze-dried lactobacillus with bifidus in a dairy (lactose)-free form. Use with intestinal distress, bowel mucous, constipation, yeast/fungal infections (after using **ADP** for 14 days), and for the intestinal side-effects of antibiotic therapy. Product does not require refrigeration. 3 tablets, TID after meals.

L-ARGININE — 700 mg per capsule. Use with free-radical problems, low growth hormone, lack of libido, fatigue, slow wound healing, male infertility, cystic fibrosis, elevated cholesterol, or liver dysfunction and degeneration. Will stimulate thymus function when used at 6000 mg or higher per day. 2 capsules, 2-TID with meals. ***Avoid during pregnancy and lactation.***

L-CARNITINE — 300 mg per capsule. Promotes energy production by enhancing fat oxidation in the cell mitochondria. Use with elevated blood fats, insulin resistance, cardiac stress, liver degeneration (cirrhosis), use with low-carbohydrate diets when the patient is unable to lose weight, muscle fatigue, senile dementia, reduced muscle mass, low sperm motility. Enhances the antioxidant effects of Vitamins C and E. 1-2 capsules, TID with meals. ***If you don't get increased energy, loss of body fat, or ketosis on 60 grams or less of carbohydrate per day, use at 4 capsules, TID with meals until you see the results you're after.***

L-GLUTAMINE — 500 mg per capsule. Use with alcoholism, sugar craving, impotence, fatigue, epilepsy, schizophrenia, mental retardation, peptic ulcers, and other gastric inflammatory problems. 2 capsules, TID with meals.

L-HISTIDINE — 600 mg per capsule. Use with rheumatoid arthritis, allergies, anemia, hypertension, and to chelate copper. 1-2 capsules, TID with meals.

LIQUID IODINE — 75 mcg of potassium iodide per drop. Use with thyroid conditions where additional iodine is required, emotional changes during the change of seasons, when the skin cracks on the hands or feet, excess or thick secretions, sinus infections, ovarian dysfunction, benign cysts and fibroids, tenderness of the area around the costal cartilage, and topically for acne, boils, and some cases of rheumatoid arthritis. 5 to 20 d daily in a glass of pure water. Increase up to 60 d per day in severe cases (short term use). ***There is a rare but potentially serious form of thyroid disease that can be made worse by iodine. Feel around your windpipe between your Adam's apple and breastbone. If you feel any swelling or bumpiness, consult a doctor before taking iodine. DON'T TAKE THIS SUPPLEMENT if you're sensitive to iodine (have trouble with seafood or diagnostic iodine).***

LIVOTRIT-PLUS — A herbal preparation based on Ayurvedic principles, with milk thistle and the trace minerals from raw sugar cane juice (The Wulzen Anti-Stiffness Factor). Use with liver disease, alcoholism, heavy-metal body burdens, and chemical or radiation damage to the liver, viruses (hepatitis, mono, EBV, CMV, etc.), and cirrhosis. Use with **Nutri-Clear** and **I.P.S.** for gastric inflammatory problems. Begin with 1 tablet, TID with meals and increase by 1 tablet every three days until a maximum of 3 tablets, TID with meals is reached. Product should always be used with **Beta-TCP** or **Beta-Plus** (to ensure that bile viscosity is thin to allow toxins a route out of the system).

LI-ZYME FORTE — Use with depression, alcoholism, fibromyalgia, thyroid hyper-function, and severe mental stress. Product is the same as **LI-Zyme**, except that each tablet contains 150 mcg of naturally occurring lithium from vegetable culture. 1-2 tablets, TID with meals.

L-PHENYLALANINE — 600 mg per capsule. Use with depression and alcoholism. 1-2 capsules, TID with meals. ***Should not be used during pregnancy, or with high blood pressure, phenylketonuria, or a pre-existing pigmented melanoma.***

L-TYROSINE — 500 mg per capsule. Use with anxiety, depression, alcoholism, drug withdrawal, and low thyroid, adrenal, or pituitary function. 1-2 capsules, TID with meals.

MCS — (Metabolic Clearing Support) A unique dietary supplement designed to balance the detoxification pathways in the liver. This supplement provides nutritional support (vitamins, sulfur-bearing amino acids, and parotid glandular) for liver detoxification. 2-4 capsules BID with meals. ***Should not be used by pregnant or lactating women.***

MEDA-STIM — An herbal/nutritional composite designed to help support low thyroid when the T-4 is normal or high and the T-3 is low. This product should be considered with **ADHS** and **G.T.A. Meda-Stim** has also been found to be effective in some cases of PMS and symptoms of mild depression that often go along with low thyroid. 1-2 capsules BID just before meals.

METHIONINE — 200-225 mg per capsule (200 mg of DL-Methionine, 20 mg of L-Lysine, 5 mg of L-Cysteine). A source of sulfur-bearing amino acids. Use with depression, Parkinson's disease, schizophrenia, skin and hair problems, biliary dysfunction, rheumatic fever, toxemia of pregnancy, and copper and other heavy-metal body burdens. 2 capsules, TID with meals.

MG-ZYME — A source of organically combined magnesium (100 mg per tablet). Use with tissue injury, muscle cramps, inflammation, PMS, cardiac stress, asthma, kidney and gall stones, as a calcium synergist, chronic fatigue, diabetes, hypoglycemia, and fibromyalgia. 4 tablets at bedtime. Increase by 1 tablet every other day until bowel intolerance occurs (loose stools).

MIXED-ASCORBATE POWDER — Contains Vitamin C in combination with calcium and magnesium ascorbate in a pH-balanced formula to improve bowel tolerance. 1 tsp in a glass of pure warm water, 2-TID.

MIXED EFAs — Contains a mixture of walnut oil, hazelnut oil, sesame oil, and apricot kernel oil. Use as a source of essential fatty acids and with ADD, ADHD, chronic fatigue, sub-acute virus, muscular dystrophy, and multiple sclerosis. 1 tsp BID.

MN-ZYME FORTE — Each tablet contains 25 mg of organically combined manganese. Use with ligament injury, disc injury, cyclic fever, virus, goiter, general immune support, insulin resistance, and as a synergist to B vitamins. 1 tablet, TID with meals.

MO-ZYME FORTE — Contains 150 mcg of naturally occurring molybdenum from vegetable culture. Use with sensitivity to MSG (use with **B6 Phosphate**), sulfites, aromatic compounds (perfume, etc.), where iron anemia doesn't respond to taking iron, or low serum uric acid (also rule out a need for folic acid and Vitamin B-12). 1 tablet, TID with meals.

MULTI-MINS — A source of organically derived minerals (a broad-spectrum formula containing both macro and micro minerals). HCl is added to facilitate the breakdown and absorption of the minerals. Use as a long-term mineral supplement, with high adrenal and/or thyroid and chronic illness. 1-2 tablets, TID with meals.

MULTI-PLUS (AQUEOUS) — An excellent, good-tasting, bioactive multiple-vitamin, multiple-mineral formula. Contains Vitamins A, C, D, E, thiamine, riboflavin, niacin, Vitamin B-6, Vitamin B-12, biotin, pantothenic acid, calcium, zinc, selenium, magnesium, copper, manganese, chromium, molybdenum and potassium. 1 tsp per day (31 teaspoon servings per bottle).

NEONATAL MULTI-GLAND — A broad-spectrum product containing both organ and gland support (contains pineal in addition to all of the other neonatal gland and organ concentrations). Use with chronic fatigue or illness, athletes under stress, for general physical or psychological stress, and as a synergist to specific gland or organ therapy. 2-3 tablets, TID with meals. *This is an excellent formula for building energy, strength, stamina, and robustness.*

NEUTROPHIL-PLUS — A blend of nutritional, glandular, and herbal components designed to stimulate phagocytosis and inhibit bacterial multiplication. Effective with upper respiratory problems to include otitis media, throat, sinus and bronchial conditions. Use with I.A.G. Adults—3-4 capsules BID between meals. Children under 12 years of age, 2-3 capsules, BID between meals or with a small amount of food. *Should not be used by pregnant or lactating females.*

NUCLEZYME FORTE — A source of RNA and DNA and synergistic factors. Use with emaciation, senility, loss of memory, brain trauma, lowered resistance to colds and viruses, as a source of B vitamins, for reduced circulation, and as a geriatric multiple-vitamin. 1 capsule, TID with meals.

NUTRI-CLEAR — A biologically active, hypoallergenic clearing formula designed to support detoxification and healing in the gastrointestinal tract, and detoxification in the liver. Use with leaky-gut syndrome, digestive inflammation (ulcers, food sensitivity), rheumatoid arthritis, and other conditions where a 5-to-7-day clearing procedure is desired. Use according to label instructions. To ensure liver clearing, always use with **Livotrit-Plus** and **Beta-TCP** or **Beta-Plus**. Use as directed on the label.

NUTRI-CLEAR/S — Use with leaky-gut syndrome, digestive inflammation (ulcers, food sensitivity), rheumatoid arthritis, and other conditions where digestive inflammation is present. This product is the same as **Nutri-Clear**, except that it uses soy protein in lieu of rice protein. Contains more protein and calories per serving than Nutri-Clear. Can be used as a clearing formula for patients who are not soy-sensitive, and for sustained periods as a daily meal replacement. Use as directed on the label.

OORGANIK-15 — Organically complexed methyl donors and acceptors (dimethyl-glycine). Enhances oxygen utilization (energy and endurance) and complexes free radicals. Use with muscular dysfunction, asthma, neuro-muscular diseases (MS, MD), athletics, and cardiac stress. 3-5 tablets, TID with meals. For endurance sports, use 5 tablets one hour before beginning the event, and 5 tablets just before beginning the event.

OPTIC-PLUS — For adjunctive supplemental support with cataracts, macular degeneration, floaters, eye strain, night blindness, and other ocular conditions *where increased inter-ocular pressure (glaucoma) has been ruled out*. 1-2 tablets, TID with meals. For floaters, add **Bio-Cyanidins** and **Cytozyme PT/HPT** (1 of each, TID.)

OSTEO-B PLUS — A source of vitamins, minerals, and other factors known to support bone growth and repair. Contains magnesium, calcium, boron, Vitamin K, silicon, manganese and B vitamins, in a base of rice bran. Use with osteoporosis, bone trauma, menopausal need for increased bone support, periodontal disease, and problems involving bone inflammation. This is also a great formula for athletes to strengthen joints and ligaments for injury prevention and quicker healing. 2 tablets, TID with meals.

PALMETTO-PLUS — A source of saw palmetto herb, magnesium, zinc, Vitamin B-6, chlorophyll, selenium, Vitamin A, lycopene, and amino acids known to support prostate function. Use with benign prostate hypertrophy. 2 capsules, TID with meals. Always use with **Flax Seed Oil** and **Liquid Iodine**. In some cases of benign prostate hypertrophy, Argizyme should also be considered with Palmetto-Plus, Flax Seed Oil, and Liquid Iodine. If you can find Pumpkin Oil, use it instead of Flax Seed Oil.

PCOH-PLUS — Each capsule contains 10 mg of policosanol (extracted from raw sugar cane), 250 mg of inositol hexaniacinate and 2.5 mg of emulsified CoQ10. PCOH-PLUS lowers cholesterol an average of 23% without the toxicity associated with cholesterol-lowering medications, increases HDL by 11%, and decreases heart attack and stroke risk by decreasing platelet aggregation. 1 capsule BID.

PHOSPHATIDYLCHOLINE — Each capsule supplies 430 mg of phosphatidylcholine and 36 mg of phosphatidyl-inositol from lecithin. Use with Alzheimer's, Parkinson's, senility, neuro-muscular disorders, nerve dysfunction, elevated blood fats, fatty liver, gall bladder symptoms, gallstones, migraine headaches, and <u>Low Adrenal</u>. 1-2 capsules, TID with meals.

PHOSPHATIDYLSERINE — Each capsule contains 100 mg of phosphatidylserine (PS). Use to improve concentration, short-term memory, energy, and mood. PS counteracts the effects of excess cortisol on the nervous system, maintains neurotransmitters, protects the myelin sheath around nerves, balances the autonomic nervous system, and increases nerve growth factor for repair of nerves damaged by excess cortisol. 2-4 caps BID.

PMT — A glandular and organ-free source of vitamins, minerals, and accessory nutrients known to support female hormone function. Product can also be used for males where a need for B vitamins, zinc, and magnesium is present, i.e., carpal tunnel syndrome. For females with PMS and other problems involving female endocrine function, use 2-3 tablets, TID with meals. For acute PMS symptoms use with **B-12/Folate Plus** and **Black Currant Seed Oil**. If the PMS involves severe hot flashes, add **Liquid Iodine**.

PNEUMA-ZYME — Source of neonatal bovine lung tissue and other factors known to support lung function. Use with upper respiratory problems, i.e., asthma, emphysema, smoker's cough, lung involvement because of adrenal and/or cardiac stress, and environmental allergy/sensitivity. 2 tablets, TID with meals.

POA-PHYTOLENS — Contains TOA-free Cat's Claw (Uncaria Tomentosa) and Phytolens, a patented extract of Lens esculata. Research indicates that Cat's Claw has antiviral, antibacterial, antioxidant, and anti-inflammatory activity. Phytolens is proven to be a potent antioxidant capable of scavenging superoxide radicals and protecting cells from nitric oxide induced inflammation. Consider using POA-Phytolens for <u>Allergies</u>, acne, fatigue, depression, PMS, and inflammatory conditions in the gastrointestinal tract (diverticulitis, colitis, gastritis, Crohn's disease). 1 cap BID/TID.

PORPHYRA-ZYME — A biologically active vegetable culture designed to chelate heavy-metals and atherosclerotic plaque. 4 tablets, TID on an empty stomach. With inflammation, use with **Intenzyme Forte**. For long-term chelation of metals or plaque, use with **Multi-Mins** or **Iron-** and **Copper-Free Multi-Mins**.

PURIFIED CHONDROITIN SULFATES — Each capsule contains 300 mg of purified chrondroitin sulfates isolated from bovine trachea. Use with disc and ligament injury, mitral valve prolapse, cartilage problems, free-radical problems, to increase the total white blood count, and in any tissue where a lack of elasticity is a known problem (vessel, artery, heart valves, etc.). 1-2 capsules, TID.

RB-ZYME — Each tablet contains 100 mcg of naturally occurring rubidium from vegetable culture. Use with cognitive problems in the elderly, chronic fatigue, and where low thyroid doesn't respond (synergist with **L-Tyrosine**). 1-2 tablets, TID with meals.

RENAL-PLUS — Contains Vitamins A, C, B-6, magnesium, neonatal organ and glandular support, as well as herbs known to support renal function and known to assist with the resolution of edema. 4 tablets, TID with meals. For acute renal problems or edema, increase to 4 tablets, 5 times a day for three days then return to 4 tablets, TID until the problem abates. *Kidney disease can be serious. If you suspect kidney infection, consult a physician.*

SELENIUM, AQUEOUS — 95 mcg of inorganic selenium per drop. Use with free-radical conditions (as an antioxidant and to control inflammation), as a synergist with Vitamin E, in Low Thyroid where the T-3 Uptake is decreased, for cardiac stress, pancreatic dysfunction, fibroids, and cysts. 1 d, TID with meals.

SE-ZYME FORTE — Each tablet contains 100 mcg of naturally occurring selenium from vegetable culture (yeast-free). Use with free-radical conditions (as an antioxidant), as a synergist with Vitamin E, reduced T-3, cardiac stress, pancreatic dysfunction, fibroids, and cysts. 1-2 tablets, TID.

SHIITAKI MUSHROOM — 500 mg of Shiitake Mushroom concentrate per capsule. Use to improve your immune function. 1-2 capsules, TID with meals. *Can be used as a source of naturally occurring and organically bound germanium.*

STAMINA CAPS — A source of L-Carnitine, Coenzyme Q-10, Octacosanol, and B vitamins. Use with athletes, muscle dysfunction, muscle injury, fatigue, and free-radical neuro-muscular diseases. 1-2 capsules, TID with meals.

THYROSTIM — A source of vitamins, minerals, glandular components, and other nutrients known to support thyroid and pituitary function. Use with Low Thyroid and Low Pituitary. 2-3 tablets, TID with meals. Always use **Thyrostim** with **Flax Seed Oil** or **Mixed EFAs**. If Low Pituitary isn't found with the Low Thyroid, add GTA at 1-2 capsules, TID. If the T-4 is normal or high and the T-3 is low, use **Meda-Stim** instead of Thyrostim.

TRI-CHOL — A unique combination of herbs, vitamins, and minerals designed to help decrease total cholesterol and triglycerides. 2 capsules, BID with breakfast and lunch.

ULTRA VIR-X — A broad-spectrum herbal and nutrient product with anti-viral and immune-stimulating properties. Has been shown to be effective with chronic and acute viral problems. Use with **IAG** and **Bio-Immunozyme Forte**. For adults, use 3-4 capsules, BID. Children under 12 years of age, use 1 capsule, BID. *Not to be used by pregnant or lactating females.*

VHP — A combination of valerian, hops and passiflora. An excellent herbal tranquilizer. Use with insomnia, nervousness, hyperactivity and hyperirritability. 1-2 capsules, TID with meals. For insomnia, use 4 capsules about 30 minutes before bedtime.

V-ZYME — Each tablet contains 20 mcg of naturally occurring vanadium from vegetable culture. Use with diabetes, elevated cholesterol, and as a synergist with chromium. 2-3 tablets, TID with meals.

ZINC, AQUEOUS — Zinc Sulfate Heptahydrate (5 mg per teaspoon) in a base of distilled water. Can be used to determine zinc deficiency as a <u>Zinc Taste Test</u> and as a zinc supplement.

ZN-ZYME FORTE — Each tablet contains 25 mg of organically combined zinc. Use with immune insufficiency, loss of sense of taste or smell, for wounds that heal slowly, acne, reduced sex drive, prostate hypertrophy, chronic yeast infections, macular degeneration, hair loss, dandruff, premature graying of the hair, white spots on the fingernails, and as a synergist with magnesium, Vitamin B-6, and chromium. 1-2 tablets, TID with meals. *Note:* If zinc is used at over 60 mg per day for over 60 days, add **CU-Zyme** at 1-2 tablets a day to prevent a zinc-copper imbalance.

Amazon Herb Company

This company makes wonderful herbal formulas made primarily of herbs from the Amazon rainforest. John Easterling, who founded the company, has taught the natives to make a living from the local plants and preserve the rainforest. The liquid formulas are spagyric extracts utilizing both the water-soluble and the alcohol-soluble aspects of each herb.

You can order directly from the Amazon Herb Company, 800-835-0850. Mention my name or *The Elements of Health* and they will take good care of you. When you order $50 or more from the company, they will make you a preferred customer and you get 30% off every order.

GRAVIZON — A powerful blend of herbs known for their support of the circulation and lymphatic system, liver, and antioxidant activity. Use for complex and chronic imbalances of the immune system that include sensitivity to the environment, chronic fatigue syndrome, fibromyalgia, Allergies, and autoimmune disorders. 1 tsp to 1 Tbsp BID/TID

LUNAZON — Balances female hormones to control PMS, normalizes menstrual cycles, and decreases tendency to yeast infections. Take 1-2 D BID/TID or 1-2 capsules BID/TID.

METABAZON — This formula supports optimal blood sugar and is useful for people with diabetes and hypoglycemia. It balances metabolic rate and thereby controls weight and improves energy. 1-2D BID/TID or 1-2 capsules BID/TID

SUMACAZON — This is a formula for chronic stress when you feel tired and worn out. Sumacazon contains Suma (commonly known as Brazilian Ginseng), Maca, Muira Puama, and Stevia. It is particularly good for people forty and older, because the herb Maca contained in this formula is very powerful support for the pituitary. Sumacazon is excellent for Low Adrenal, Blood Sugar Problems, Low Pituitary, Female Hormonal, and Male Hormonal. Take 1-2 D BID or TID or 1-2 capsules BID or TID.

WARRIOR — This formula contains traditional herbs from Chinese medicine as well as herbs from the Amazon. The rainforest herbs in Warrior are Muira Puama, Catuaba, and Sarsaparilla. These are blended with the Shaolin Temple martial arts formula of Wild Yam root, Astragalus, Rehmannia, Atractylodes, Tangerine Peel, Costas Root, Glycyrrhiza, Dong Quai, Fennel, and Aquilaria. Warrior is excellent for Low Adrenal and Blood Sugar Problems. It builds strength and robustness and helps you handle stress better. This is a great formula for athletes. Take 1-2 D BID or TID or 1-2 capsules BID or TID.

UNA DE GATO — This herb is the inner bark of a vine and is highly revered by native peoples in the Amazon. It's a very versatile herb. In this workbook, I have recommended it as an immune regulator. It can be used to clear up infections in the gut (dysbiosis), balance the autonomic nervous system, for general detoxification, to improve digestion and absorption, heal the gut lining from leaky-gut syndrome, and decrease inflammation (colitis, arthritis, and fibromyalgia). It is also wonderful for chronic fatigue syndrome and allergies. Take 1-2 D BID or TID or 1-2 capsules BID or TID.

Dragon River

Dragon River makes many fine herbal tinctures. In this workbook, I have focused on a formula I feel is the most effective I've ever used to treat people with health problems due to chronic stress and the inability to relax.

Parasympa is an herbal tincture (liquid extract) made of **Damiana**, **Kava Kava**, and **Oat Seed**. The oat seed is collected when it is still green. When the still-green oat seed is squeezed between your fingers, a rich milky liquid comes out. Both of these herbs are traditionally used to help people with nervous exhaustion, or as it's referred to these days, chronic fatigue syndrome. Parasympa increases the tone of the parasympathetic nervous system. It helps people relax. I consider it the first stage of getting someone well when they are unable to relax or suffer from chronic stress. Parasympa is available from from *The Elements of Health*, 866-563-4256, or online at www.theelementsofhealth.com.

These herbs are reputed to be aphrodisiacs. Sexual response is mostly controlled by the parasympathetic nervous system. If you're in a High Autonomic (Sympathetic Dominant) state, it's very difficult to get in the mood sexually. If your body is stuck in a fight-or-flight response, sex isn't really considered by your body to be a high priority. It's not important for immediate survival. So your body can't get turned on because the circuit for getting turned on is shut off. Getting your autonomic nervous system balanced opens up that circuit and your body can respond sexually.

You may feel very tired for the first 3-7 days. The more you've depleted your body from stress, the longer and more profoundly you will feel tired. After that, your energy will build, but it will be relaxed, real energy. You will know you're on the right track, because after a few days you will start to feel more rested when you wake up in the morning.

Often with very chronic stress and over-stimulation, you will experience nervous exhaustion. Anytime there has been severe and/or chronic stress in your life and you experience fatigue or even exhaustion, take Parasympa. It is the most consistently useful remedy for stress I have ever used. I usually have people take two droppers-full in water three times a day for six weeks, then take Parasympa afterwards as needed.

Some people end up doing very well taking a little Parasympa on a regular basis. Long-term, the dosage is best regulated based on how you feel. Ideally, you will be relaxed and more energetic. You will also handle stressful situations more easily. The ongoing need for this remedy is usually due to either being under ongoing stress or because of a genetic tendency to being High Autonomic (sympathetic dominant).

Take 2D TID in some water for six weeks to reset your system, and then as needed.

KAL

NUTRITIONAL YEAST — This food is a very concentrated source of B vitamins, zinc, chromium, selenium, phosphorus, and amino acids. They are present in their natural forms. This is a great supplement for energy and to balance blood sugar. Most health food stores carry the KAL brand. If you can't find Nutritional Yeast locally, it is also available from *The Elements of Health*.

Standard Process Labs

Standard Process products can be ordered from *The Elements of Health*, 866-563-4256, or online at www.theelementsofhealth.com, or directly from doctors endorsing and incorporating the *choosing* HEALTH system.

CHOLACOL II — Contains Montmorillonite and bile salts. For improving absorption, take 4 tablets about 15 minutes before each meal for two weeks (this takes two bottles). For mild food poisoning, take 2-4 tablets every half hour until you get relief. Then go to every hour; if you're still feeling good, go to every two hours. At that point take 3 QID for a few days to make sure the problem doesn't sneak up on you. This is very useful for people who have trouble maintaining their weight, or who take supplements but don't seem to get any benefit from them. A sure sign of needing Cholacol II is feeling hungry, looking into the refrigerator, and not really knowing what you want to eat.

DI-SODIUM PHOSPHATE — This is used for cleansing programs. It has a mild laxative effect. One to four capsules can be used at bedtime as a mild laxative.

Yerba Prima

Wonderful herbal formulas. Yerba Prima products can be purchased at health food stores or from *The Elements of Health*.

HYDRATED BENTONITE — Liquid Bentonite is less convenient than Cholacol II to take, but does work better. For improving absorption take 1-2 tablespoons BID or TID in dilute apple cider (preferably raw and unfiltered). For mild food poisoning, you can take at the frequency outlined for Cholacol II. Start with a teaspoon and work up to the larger dosage. Sometimes people get a little constipated when they first start taking Liquid Bentonite, if they don't drink enough water and don't give themselves a chance to get used to it. I often give this to people for up to twelve weeks at a time with a bulking agent like Colon Plus powder (BRC).

KALENITE — This formula cleanses the intestinal tract, liver/gall bladder, and lymphatic system. It is stronger than **Herbal Guard**, yet can be used on an ongoing basis for very deep detoxification. 1-6 tablets BID

MEN'S REBUILD INTERNAL CLEANSING SYSTEM — This is basically the men's version. This comes as a boxed set of bottles of Colon Care, Herbal Guard, and Men's Rebuild. Colon Care, Herbal Guard, and Men's Rebuild are also available individually.

WOMEN'S RENEW INTERNAL CLEANSING SYSTEM — This is a very effective and gentle cleanse. Most cleansing programs get fairly complicated and are hard to do for people with a busy schedule. This cleanse couldn't be easier. Take capsules as directed morning and night. This comes as a boxed set of bottles of Colon Care, Herbal Guard, and Women's Renew. **Colon Care**, **Herbal Guard**, and **Woman's Renew** are also available individually.

Note: Women's Renew and Men's Rebuild purchased from the health food store contain Senna and Cascara Sagrada, whereas Women's Renew and Men's Rebuild from *The Elements of Health* do not. These herbs are useful to stimulate regularity, but for some people these can be too strong and cause abdominal pain.

How To Find Functional Medicine Doctors

What is a Doctor?

A doctor is someone who has been trained and is licensed to diagnose. Doctors who meet these criteria are also called primary physicians. They determine what's going on, suggest what needs to be done, and recommend who best can get the job done for you.

Medicine is a generic term. Medicine is the study and practice of health care with the application of therapies to eliminate disease and restore health. No one kind of doctor has a corner on the market. Whatever will best get the job done for you is the right kind of medicine for you. It's not about being dogmatic; it's about being pragmatic.

Primary Physicians		
Title	**Type of Medicine**	**Nature of Practice**
Doctor of Chiropractic (DC)	Chiropractic	Correcting the nervous system to eliminate nerve interference, thereby allowing full expression of the body's innate intelligence to heal. DCs often incorporate nutrition, herbs, acupuncture, and other natural therapies to complement care.
Doctor of Osteopathy (DO)	Osteopathic	Correcting the soft tissues of the body so there is complete and unrestricted circulation of oxygen, nutrients, and energy to allow healing. License includes the use of drugs, surgery, nutrition, and some DOs may use other natural therapies as well.
Homeopathic Medical Doctor (MD(H))	Homeopathic	Using extremely minute doses of plant, animal, and mineral substances to stimulate a healing response in the body. Homeopaths often use other therapies to complement the use of homeopathy.
Medical Doctor (MD)	Allopathic	Using drugs and surgery to correct or manage disease. Many MDs now add nutrition, lifestyle therapies, and a host of other natural therapies to their care.
Naturopathic Medical Doctor (NMD) or Naturopathic Doctor (ND)	Naturopathic	Using natural elements (food, water, air, nutrients, herbs) and natural factors (exercise, rest, hygiene, stress management, physical therapies (including manipulation) to restore the body's inherent capacity to heal and regulate itself. May include homeopathy, acupuncture, and the use of prescription medicines in some states.
Oriental Medical Doctor (OMD)	Oriental Medicine or Traditional Chinese Medicine (TCM)	Using natural elements, natural factors (including herbs), and acupuncture to restore balance and harmony to qi (body energy) thereby, allow the body to heal and regulate itself.

What is a Functional Medicine Doctor?

A functional medicine doctor is any primary physician who is trained and focused in diagnosing and treating functional illnesses. A functional medicine doctor uses functional medicine to restore health by restoring function.

The following organizations, each detailed on the following pages, can put you in touch with doctors who practice functional medicine:

- **International College of Applied Kinesiology (ICAK)**
- **International Foundation for Nutrition and Health (IFNH)**
- **Price-Pottenger Nutrition Foundation (PPNF)**
- **The Weston A. Price Founcation (WAPF)**

International College of Applied Kinesiology (ICAK)

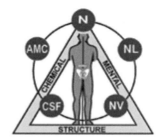

Phone:	913-384-5336
Fax:	913-384-5112
Address:	6405 Metcalf Ave, Suite 503
	Shawnee Mission, KS 66202-3929
E-mail:	info@icakusa.com
Website:	www.icakusa.com (online referral directory)

Applied Kinesiology (AK) is a form of diagnosis that uses muscle testing to determine how your body functions. AK is used not only to find the exact functional diagnosis, but also the best therapy for your unique needs. The focus of AK is to treat the five factors regulating your health in order to restore balance to the triad of health.

The Five Factors Regulating Your Health According to AK

Abbreviation	Name	Function
N	Nerve	Nervous System (includes nutrition)
NL	Neurolymphatic	Lymphatic system
NV	Neurovascular	Vascular system
CSF	Cerebrospinal Fluid	Craniosacral mechanism (controls central nervous system)
AMC	Acupuncture Meridian Connector	Meridian system (balancing Chi energy and acupuncture)

In general, an applied kinesiologist finds a muscle that tests weak and then attempts to determine why that muscle is not functioning properly. This leads to the underlying dysfunction that's present. The applied kinesiologist then determines the "best fit" therapy based on testing your body's response to a wide array of potential therapies drawn from all of the healing arts. After treatment, AK can be used to determine your response to the therapy and whether or not your function has improved.

choosing HEALTH

Muscle testing is only part of the applied kinesiology-focused functional medicine approach. History, physical exams, laboratory, and other specialty exams drawn from medicine are all used together to understand fully the complete picture of your health. Very accurate diagnosis of the way your body functions, clear understanding of the interplay between all parts of your body systems, and exact knowledge of what needs to be done to restore optimal body function are the forte of AK.

Dr. George Goodheart founded applied kinesiology in 1964. The International College of Applied Kinesiology was founded in 1976 by a group of doctors who had been teaching AK. The purpose of the College is to promote research and the teaching of AK. It is a professional association dedicated to bringing together doctors and students with common interests and goals. It takes many hundreds of hours of study and years of practice to perfect the multitude of diagnostic techniques developed in AK.

Main Therapies From The Healing Arts Incorporated Into AK

Therapy	Origins	Effect
Chiropractic	Chiropractic	Eliminates nerve interference; enhances function and organization of the nervous system; restores normal mechanics to body joints.
Craniosacral	Osteopathy	Eliminates nerve interference; enhances function and organization of the nervous system; restores mechanics.
Acupuncture	Oriental medicine	Restores energy and balance to Chi (body energy); balances the nervous system.
Muscle and Reflex Therapies	All healing arts	Improves circulation of blood and lymph; helps to reorganize the nervous system; increases range of motion.
Clinical Nutrition	All healing arts	Provides raw materials for your body to function; normalizes body chemistry; compensates for genetic weaknesses and toxic environment.
Herbal Medicine & Homeopathy	All healing arts (primarily naturopathy)	Detoxifies the body from the effects of toxic environment; eliminates infections; provides nutrients; restores self-regulation of the body.
Neuroemotional Technique	Integration of the healing arts	Repatterns limiting beliefs created from conditioning experiences (primarily in early life); restores emotional balance and resilience.

Chiropractic (N)

Look well to the spine for the cause of disease. ~ Hippocrates

Your spine is the circuit board for your nervous system. The nerves that exit at the level of each vertebra of your spine travel to and innervate every gland, organ, muscle, and indeed, every part of your body. These nerves integrate, organize, and regulate all living processes.

Every vertebra that makes up your spine is like a circuit breaker, and your spine, as a whole, makes up the circuit breaker box. If there is a tripped circuit breaker in your house, whatever that circuit goes to isn't going to work — there's no electricity, no energy getting there. Your body is just like that — to get any part of your body to work it has to at least get nerve supply (electricity) from the nerves exiting the spine.

These tripped circuit breakers in your body are called subluxations. Chiropractic resolves subluxations through an adjustment to the spine and other joints in your body, thereby eliminating nerve interference. Without nerve interference, your body's innate intelligence is fully expressed and the inherent ability of your body to be self-healing and self-regulating is present.

Craniosacral Therapy (CSF)

Osteopathic craniosacral therapy reinforces and restores motion to the spine, pelvis, and skull. Complementary to chiropractic care, craniosacral therapy also helps eliminate nerve interference and nurtures full nerve expression. Craniosacral therapy increases motion and suppleness to the spine. Often, when chiropractic care is making useful but temporary changes, craniosacral therapy is needed.

Acupuncture (AMC)

Chinese medicine, of which acupuncture is a part, is a complete system of health care that has existed for over two thousand years. The intention of Chinese medicine is to restore harmony to yin and yang, balance to the five elements (fire, earth, metal, water, and wood), bring poise and freedom to the flow of Qi (chi) through the meridian pathways of the body, allow the natural flow of the elements within your body in accord with the seasons, and strength to Jing (primordial body energy), Qi, and Shen (spirit).

Chinese medicine has traditionally used bone-setting (essentially chiropractic care), diet, stress, and lifestyle management, herbal medicine, internal exercise like Tai Chi and Chi Kung, and meridian therapy (which includes acupuncture).

Modern acupuncture uses an ohmmeter to measure the energy in each of your twelve major meridians. This information is entered into a computer where the information is processed and graphed. Follow-up exams will show the changes taking place in your meridian system due to treatment. Needles aren't required. Tapping, heat, cold, rubbing, gentle electrical stimulation, and even laser can be used to balance the flow of Qi through the meridians.

Muscle and Reflex Therapies (NL and NV)

Applied Kinesiology (AK) incorporates muscle and reflex therapies. Neurovascular reflex therapies improve blood flow, neurolymphatic reflexes from osteopathy improve lymphatic drainage and hand, foot, and skin reflexes restore nerve function.

To restore integrity to the muscles of your body, AK draws from the myofascial techniques of Rolfing, strain-counterstrain techniques of Osteopathy, and trigger-point techniques from traditional (Allopathic) medicine. Additionally AK utilizes muscle techniques unique to it such as reactive and frozen muscle patterns.

Clinical Nutrition (N)

Your food shall be your medicine and your medicine shall be your food.   ~ Hippocrates

Nutrition is necessary to support body growth and repair and to sustain metabolism. Your body function cannot be maintained and even your genetic potential cannot be expressed without necessary nutrients. Dietary recommendations are the foundation of clinical nutrition, but you may also need supplementation. Many factors cause the need for supplements in your diet: pollution, stress, processing of foods and food additives, and foods grown on depleted soils. Counseling regarding your unique dietary needs greatly complements the nutritional supplementation.

Clinical nutrition recommendations are determined by integrating information from your history, exam findings, lab findings, and applied kinesiology.

Herbal Medicine and Homeopathy (N)

Herbs are most important for detoxification and eliminating infections. Well-chosen herb or herb formulas can address your genetic constitution, strengthening your body as a whole, and preventing you from developing illnesses associated with your genetic makeup.

Very small, even infinitesimal dilutions of plant, mineral, and animal substances are used in homeopathy to stimulate a healing response. Homeopathy can be very helpful to resolve residual problems from a past trauma or infection.

Neuroemotional Technique (N)

We respond to the world around us and process our experiences based on our conditioning. Often the conditioning we learned when we were very young and still use on a daily basis no longer serves us well.

There are a number of techniques used in AK, for the mental/emotional side of the Triad of Health. Not all doctors using applied kinesiology use NET, but I have included it here because NET is a technique developed from the tools of AK, and many doctors who use AK also use NET.

Through the use of neuro-emotional technique (NET), we can determine how stress is affecting you physically and repattern the conditioning so it no longer affects you. Using NET is a remarkably fast, painless, exciting, and efficient approach to understanding and resolving the conditioned responses causing you stress.

NET is used to correct Neuro-Emotional Complexes (NECs). These conditioned responses cause physical and/or emotional distress and can result in illness. Conditioned responses can also be the basis of limiting beliefs that restrict the freedom you have to express yourself fully in any given situation in day-to-day life. I have seen profound changes in people's lives when NECs are cleared up.

International Foundation for Nutrition and Health (IFNH)

Phone: 858-488-8932
Fax: 858-488-2566
Address: 3963 Mission Boulevard, San Diego, CA 92109
Email: ifnh@ifnh.org
Website: www.ifnh.org

The International Foundation for Nutrition and Health trains doctors in functional medicine and can provide a referral for doctors who are members of the organization. Doctors associated with this group are trained in using the acoustic cardiograph. This instrument graphs the heart sounds from the four heart valves.

Doctors trained in reading graphs from the acoustic cardiograph can derive an amazing amount of information about how your body is working. These graphs can provide information about your heart, liver, gall bladder, digestion, lung function, kidneys, muscles, nerves, vitamins and minerals, and essential fatty acids. The graphs also tell about stress and how your adrenal glands function.

Your health and the improvement in your body's function can be monitored on an ongoing basis with use of the acoustic cardiograph. It is one of the most important tools in my office. Using the acoustic cardiograph, I know what needs to be fixed and if I don't fix whatever needs fixing, it's right there on the graph until I get the job done!

Price-Pottenger Nutrition Foundation (PPN)

Phone: 800-366-3748 or 619-462-7600
Fax: 619-433-3136
Address: P.O. Box 2614, La Mesa, CA 91943-2614
Email   info@price-pottenger.org
Website: www.price-pottenger.org

The Price-Pottenger Foundation provides a directory of doctors trained in functional medicine and provides information, books and videos on diet, nutrition, stress management, and healthy lifestyle. They're a tremendous resource.

In particular, they have the books of Drs. Price and Pottenger available. They also have books, including cookbooks, to help you incorporate the concepts and principles from Dr. Price's and Dr. Pottenger's books into your diet.

The Weston A. Price Foundation (WAPF)

Phone: 202-333-HEAL (4325)
Address: PMB 106-380, 4200 Wisconsin Avenue, NW, Washington, DC 20016
Email: westonaprice@msn.com
Website: www.westonaprice.org

This foundation does a wonderful job promoting the concepts of Weston Price and is a good resource for dietary information and access to organic foods, etc. They also have fantastic articles on their website.

About Dr. Force

Mark Force, D.C.
The Elements of Health

7500 East Pinnacle Peak Road, Suite A-207
Scottsdale, Arizona 85255
Phone: 480-563-4256
Fax: 480-563-4269
E-mail: mforcedc@earthlink.net
Website: www.theelementsofhealth.com

Services

- Chiropractic
- Acupuncture
- Clinical Nutrition
- **Applied Kinesiology**
- Craniosacral Therapy
- Neuro-emotional Technique
- Exams, reports of findings, and treatment
- Review of records and recommendations
- Lab kits and direct lab testing
- Consulting services
- Second opinions
- Seminars

Professional Contributions

Teach acupuncture, applied kinesiology, clinical nutrition, and diagnosis to physicians and student physicians. Conduct clinical research for Biotics Research Labs in the development of nutritional formulations and assessment of the efficacy of those formulations.

Professional Organizations

- Diplomate and Certified Instructor, International College of Applied Kinesiology (ICAK)
- Advanced Fellow and Instructor, International Academy of Medical Acupuncture (FIAMA)
- Member, International Foundation for Nutrition and Health (IFNH)
- Price-Pottenger Nutrition Foundation (PPNF)

Published Papers

- *Tonic Labyrinthine Reflexes and Center of Gravity: Preliminary Observations,* published in the Collected Papers of the International College of Applied Kinesiology (ICAK), 1988

- *Use of Myopulse in the Correction of Myofascial Adhesions,* published in the Collected Papers of the ICAK, 1988

- *A Manual for Metabolic/Nutritional Evaluation of the SMA/25, CBC with Differential and Related Tests*; Balancing Body Chemistry with Nutrition; Cannonsburg, MI; technical contributor, 1989

- *Nutritional Protocols,* Balancing Body Chemistry with Nutrition; Cannonsburg, MI; technical contributor, 1992

- *On the Use of Glandular Preparations in Clinical Practice,* Selected Papers of the International College of Applied Kinesiology; 1994

- *Inhibition of Enteric Parasites by Emulsified Oil of Oregano in vivo,* M. Force et al, Phytotherapy Research, 14, 213-214 (2000); Index Medicus listed.

Bibliography

Functional Selfcare and Choosing Health

Mental and Elemental Nutrients (Carl Pfeiffer, MD, PhD; Keats, 1976)

Predictive Medicine (Cheraskin, E., MD, Ringsdorf, W.M. Jr., DMD; Keats, 1973).

Diet and Disease (Cheraskin, E., MD, Ringsdorf, W.M. Jr., DMD and Clark, J.W., DDS; Keats, 1968)

Healing And The Mind (Bill Moyer, Doubleday, New York, 1993)

Your Health Under Siege (Jeffrey Bland, PhD; Stephen Greene Press; Brattleboro, Vermont; 1981)

The Elements of Health

Breathing

Conscious Breathing (Gay Hendricks, Bantam, 1995); available from 800-688-0772 or www.hendricks.com.

Water

Your Bodies' Many Cries for Water (Batmanghelidj, F., MD, Global Health Solutions, 1992) can be ordered from 800-759-3999, www.watercure.com (fascinating articles and resources)

Water: The Shocking Truth That Can Save Your Life (Paul Bragg, Health Science, 1999); all of Paul Bragg's inspiring books are available from 800-446-1990 or www.bragg.com.

Salt

Seasalt's Hidden Powers (Jacques de Langre, PhD; Happiness Press, 1992; available from The Grain and Salt Society, 800-867-7258, www.celtic-seasalt.com.

Foundation Diet

Nutrition and Physical Degeneration (Weston Price, DDS; Keats, 1989); available from Price-Pottenger Nutrition Foundation (PPNF), (800) 366-3748 or (619) 462-7600, www.price-pottenger.org.

Pottenger's Cats: A Study In Nutrition (Francis Pottenger, MD; Price-Pottenger Nutrition Foundation, San Diego, 1995); also available from Price-Pottenger Nutrition Foundation (PPNF).

Raw Energy (Leslie and Susannah Kenton, Warner Books, New York, 1984).

Empty Harvest (Bernard Jensen and Mark Anderson, Avery Publishing; Garden City Park, NY; 1990).

Non-Toxic Environment

Chemical Time Bomb (Doris Rapp, MD; Bantam, New York, 1996); Dr. Rapp does brilliant work for kids with allergies and behavioral problems. Other highly recommended books by Dr. Rapp also available from 716-875-0398 or www.drrapp.com.

Bibliography (continued)

The Elements of Health (continued)

Detoxification and Fasting

Inner Cleansing (Carlson Wade, Parker Publishing; Englewood Cliffs, NJ; 1992).

The Miracle of Fasting (Paul Bragg, ND; Health Science, 1999); available from 800-446-1990 or www.bragg.com.

How To Keep Slim, Healthy, and Young with Juice Fasting (Paavo Airola, ND; Health Plus Publishing, 1971); this and Dr. Airola's other books are available from 503-625-0589 or www.healthpluspublishers.com.

Exercise

Aerobic

Challenge Yourself at Any Age (Clarence Bass, Clarence Bass's Ripped; 1999; order from 505-266-5858. Articles online at www.cbass.com.

Anaerobic

Challenge Yourself at Any Age (Clarence Bass, Clarence Bass's Ripped; 1999; order from 505-266-5858. Articles online at www.cbass.com.

Getting Stronger (Bill Pearl, Shelter Publications; Bolinas, CA; 1986), available from 541-535-3363 or www.billpearl.com.

Power to the People (Pavel Tsatsouline, Dragon Door, 1999; to order 800-899-5111, articles online at www.dragondoor.com.

Renegade Training for Football (Coach Davies, Dragon Door); to order 800-899-5111, articles online at www.dragondoor.com.

The Russian Kettlebell Challenge (Pavel Tsatsouline, Dragon Door, 2000).

From Russia With Tough Love (Pavel Tsatsouline, Dragon Door, 2002).

Flexibility

Yoga: The Iyengar Way (Silva, Mira, & Shiyam Mehta; Knopf, New York, 1990).

Stretching for Everyday Fitness (Bob Anderson, Shelter Publications, 2000; order from Stretching Online, 800-333-1307, www.stretching.com.

How to Use Yoga (Mira Mehta, Rodmell Press, 1998).

Relax Into Stretch (Pavel Tsatsouline, Dragon Door; to order 800-899-5111, articles online at www.dragondoor.com.

Superjoints (Pavel Tsatsouline, Dragon Door; to order 800-899-5111, articles online at www.dragondoor.com.

Bibliography (continued)

Exercise (continued)

Neuromuscular

Mind Body Mastery (Dan Millman, New World Library, 1999); available from www.danmillman.com.

Energetic

Ancient Secrets of the Fountain of Youth (Peter Kelder, New York, Doubleday, 1998), book set and an accompanying video are available from Harbor Press, 253-851-5190.

Yoga: The Iyengar Way (Silva, Mira, & Shiyam Mehta; Knopf, New York, 1990).

The Way of Qigong (Ken Cohen, Ballantine, 1999).

The Way of Energy (Lam Kan Chuen, Fireside, 1991).

Step-by-Step Tai Chi (Lam Kan Chuen, Fireside, 1994).

Sleep, Rest and Relaxation

The Promise of Sleep (William Dement, Delacorte, New York, 1999).

Being Present and Doing Nothing

How to Think Like Leonardo da Vinci (Michael Gelb, Delacorte Press, New York, 1998).

Touching (Ashley Montague, Harper, New York, 1971).

The Pleasure Zone (Stella Resnick, Ph.D, Conari Press, Berkeley, 1997).

Fear of Life (Alexander Lowen, MD; Collier Books, New York, 1980).

Toward a Psychology of Being (Abraham Maslow, John Wiley and Sons, New York, 1999).

Radiance: Breathwork, Movement & Body-Centered Psychotherapy (Gay & Kathlyn Hendricks, Wingbow Press, Berkeley, 1991).

Moderation

Handbook To Higher Consciousness (Ken Keyes, Living Love Publications; Coos Bay, Oregon; 1975).

Gathering Power Through Insight and Love (Ken Keyes, Living Love Publications; Coos Bay, Oregon; 1987).

Man's Search For Meaning (Viktor Frankl, Touchstone, New York, 1984).

The Meditations (Marcus Aurelius, Modern Library, 2002).

An Open Heart: Practicing Compassion in Everyday Life (Dalai Lama, Little Brown & Co., 2001).

Bibliography (continued)

Recreation (Play)

Joy: The Surrender to the Body and to Life (Alexander Lowen, MD; Arkana (a division of Penguin), New York, 1995).

Deep Play (Diane Ackerman, Random House, New York, 1999).

Healthy Pleasures (Robert Ornstein, PhD, and David Sobel, MD; Addison-Wesley, New York, 1989).

The Pleasure Connection (Deva Beck, RN and James Beck, RN; Synthesis Press, San Marcos, CA; 1987).

Flow (Mihaly Csikzentmihalyi, Harper Perennial, New York, 1994).

At The Speed Of Life (Gay Hendricks, PhD and Kathlyn Hendricks, PhD; Bantam, New York, 1990).

Meditation, Contemplation and Prayer

The Relaxation Response (Herbert Benson, MD, Avon Books, New York, 1975); available from The Mind Body Medical Institute, 866-509-0732, www.mbmi.com.

The Heartmath Solution (Doc Childre and Howard Martin, Harper, San Francisco, 1999); articles, research, books and tapes on validated stress management techniques, 800-450-9111, www.heartmath.com.

Breath by Breath (Larry Rosenberg, Shambala, Boston, 1999).

The Contemplative Journey (Father Thomas Keating, Sounds True, Boulder, CO), audiotape set, 800-333-9185, www.soundstrue.com.

The Present Moment (Thich Nhat Hanh, Sounds True, Boulder, CO), audiotape set, 800-333-9185, www.soundstrue.com.

Putting on the Mind of Christ (Jim Marion, Hampton Roads, 2000).

The Direct Path: Creating A Journey To The Divine Through The Worlds Traditions (Andrew Harvey, Broadway Books, 2001).

Living Presence: A Sufi Way to Mindfulness & the Essential Self (Kabir Edmund Helminski; Jeremy P. Tarche/Perigree (a division of Putnam), New York, 1992).

The Science of Mind (Ernest Holmes, J. P. Tarcher, 1998).

Pure Unlimited Love: An Eternal Creative Force and Blessing Taught by All Religions (Sir John Templeton, Templeton Foundation, 2000).

Relationships

Conscious Loving (Gay Hendricks, Ph.D. and Kathlyn Hendricks, Ph.D.; Bantam, New York, 1990); available from 800-688-0772 or www.hendricks.com.

The Conscious Heart (Gay Hendricks, PhD and Kathlyn Hendricks, PhD; New York, Bantam, 1997).

Intimate Communion (David Deida, Health Communications, 1995); David Deida has a number of brilliant books and tapes available from 888-626-9662 or www.deida.com.

Bibliography (continued)

Sleep, Rest and Relaxation (continued)

Mission and Purpose

Think and Grow Rich (Napoleon Hill); also available as an audiotape set from Nigtingale Conant, 800-525-9000, www.nightingale.com.

Napoleon Hill's Keys to Success (Napoleon Hill), also available as an audiotape set, the *Science of Personal Achievement* from Nightingale Conant, 800-525-9000, www.nightingale.com.

Contribution

Laws Of Inner Wealth (Sir John Templeton), audiotape set from Nightingale Conant, 800-525-9000, www.nightingale.com.

The Health Graph, Using Home Tests, and Using Lab Tests

Trace Elements, Hair Analysis and Nutrition (Passwater, Richard A., PhD & Cranton, Elmer M., MD, (Keats Publishing, Inc., 1983).

Lectures of Dr. Royal Lee, Volume I (Mark R Anderson, Selene River Press, Inc.; 1988).

Nutritional Biochemistry and Metabolism (Linder, Maria C., PhD; Elsevier Science Publishing Company, Inc.; 1991).

The Nutritional Protocol Manual (Downey, Dolores S., Editor, Balancing Body Chemistry with Nutrition, 1996).

More Than Just A Bunch of Numbers — Making Sense of Blood Chemistry Results (Dolores Downey, Editor; Balancing Body Chemistry with Nutrition, 1984).

Zinc and Other Micro-Nutrients (Carl Pfeiffer, MD; Keats, 1978).

How to Get Well (Paavo Airola, ND; Health Plus Publishers, 1974).

Applied Kinesiology (David Walther, DC; Systems DC, Pueblo, CO, 1988-2000).

Food Is Your Best Medicine (Henry Bieler, MD; Random House, New York, 1965).

Medical Applications of Clinical Nutrition (Jeffrey Bland, PhD; Keats, 1983).

Vitamin News (Lee, Royal, DDS, Vitamin Products Company, 1942).

Applied Protomorphology (Royal Lee, DDS; Standard Process Laboratories, 1952).

Compiled Notes on Clinical Nutritional Products (Walter Schmitt, DC; David Barmore Productions, New York, 1990).

Protomorphology (Royal Lee and William Hanson, W.A. Krueger Co., Wisconsin, 1947).

Psycho-Dietetics (E. Cheraskin, MD, DMD and W. M. Ringsdorf, DMD, Bantam, New York, 1974).

Fats That Heal Fats That Kill (Udo Erasmus, Alive Books, Burnaby, BC, Canada; 1993).

Bibliography *(continued)*

The Health Graph, Using Home Tests, and Using Lab Tests *(continued)*

Harper's Biochemistry (Robert Murray, Daryl Granner, Peter Mayes, Victor Rodwell; Appleton & Lange; Stamford, CT; 1996).

Omega 3 Oils (Donald Rudin, MD; Avery Publishing Group, 1996).

Zinc and Other Micro-Nutrients (Carl Pfeiffer, PhD, MD; Keats, 1978).

Metabolic Aspects of Health: Nutritional Elements in Health and Disease (Karl Schutte, PhD & John Myers, MD, Discovery Press, California, 1979).

The Real Truth About Vitamins And Antioxidants (Judith Decava, Brentwood Academic Press; Colombus, Georgia; 1996).

Body Chemistry in Health and Disease (Melvin Page, DDS; The Page Foundation, St. Petersburg Beach, FL; 2001).

Applied Nutrition (Harold Hawkins, DDS; Mojave Books, 1977).

Textbook of Nutritional Medicine (Melvyn Werbach, MD; Thirdline Press, 1999).

Foundations of Nutritional Medicine (Melvyn Werbach, MD; Thirdline Press, 1997).

Stress and Life

The Stress of Life (Hans Selye, MD; McGraw-Hill Professional Publishing, 1978)

Stress without Distress (Hans Selye, MD; New American Library, 1991)

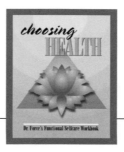

Name: _____ Date ___/___/___ Test #: ___

Digestion Problems

1	Bad breath	0	1	2	3
2	Loss of appetite for high-protein foods (meat, etc.)	0	1	2	3
3	Eating relieves an acid stomach	0	1	2	3
4	Gas shortly after eating	0	1	2	3
5	Indigestion ½-1 hour after eating	0	1	2	3
6	Difficulty digesting fruits & vegetables; undigested food in stool	0	1	2	3
7	Acid or spicy foods upset stomach	0	1	2	3

Liver/Gall Bladder

8	Lower bowel gas and/or bloating several hours after eating	0	1	2	3
9	Feet burn	0	1	2	3
10	Whites of eyes (sclera) yellow	0	1	2	3
11	Dry skin; itchy skin; skin peels on feet	0	1	2	3
12	Brown spots or bronzing of skin	0	1	2	3
13	Bitter metallic taste in mouth	0	1	2	3
14	Blurred vision	0	1	2	3
15	Headache over eyes	0	1	2	3
16	Feel nauseous, get queasy and/or gag easily	0	1	2	3
17	Color of stools light brown or yellow	0	1	2	3
18	Greasy or high-fat foods cause distress	0	1	2	3
19	Pain between shoulder blades	0	1	2	3
20	Dark circles under eyes	0	1	2	3
21	Acid breath	0	1	2	3
22	History of gall bladder attacks or gall bladder removed	N	—	—	Y
23	Appetite reduced	0	1	2	3

Large Intestine

24	Coated tongue or fuzzy debris on tongue	0	1	2	3
25	Pass large amounts of foul-smelling gas	0	1	2	3
26	Irritable bowel or mucous colitis	0	1	2	3
27	Alternating constipation and diarrhea	0	1	2	3
28	Bowel movements painful or difficult; constipation	0	1	2	3
29	Burning or itching anus	0	1	2	3

Allergies

30	Head congestion/sinus fullness	0	1	2	3
31	Sneezing attacks	0	1	2	3
32	Nightmares and bad dreams	0	1	2	3
33	Milk products and/or wheat products cause distress	0	1	2	3
34	Eyes and nose watery	0	1	2	3
35	Eyes swollen and puffy	0	1	2	3
36	Pulse speeds after meals and/or heart pounds after retiring	0	1	2	3

Immune System

37	Chronic or recurrent infections	0	1	2	3
38	Constant lung congestion	0	1	2	3
39	Heal slowly from infections	0	1	2	3
40	Autoimmune disease (rheumatoid arthritis, MS, etc.)	0	1	2	3
41	Chronic fatigue syndrome and/or fibromyalgia syndrome	0	1	2	3

Blood Sugar Problems

		0	1	2	3
42	Crave sugar, sodas, or coffee in mid-morning or early afternoon	0	1	2	3
43	Hungry between meals, excessive appetite, or always hungry	0	1	2	3
44	Eating sweets upsets	0	1	2	3
45	Eat compulsively when nervous, anxious, or stressed	0	1	2	3
46	Irritable before meals	0	1	2	3
47	Shaky, weak, irritable, or light-headed between meals	0	1	2	3
48	Fatigue; eating relieves	0	1	2	3
49	Heart palpitates if meals are missed/delayed	0	1	2	3
50	Wake at night; hard to get back to sleep	0	1	2	3
51	Frequent unrealistic fears or worries	0	1	2	3
52	Often have to eat in the middle of the night	0	1	2	3
53	Often hard to concentrate or have trouble remembering things	0	1	2	3
54	Become anxious without reason	0	1	2	3
55	Excessively weak for no apparent reason	0	1	2	3
56	Often moody or depressed	0	1	2	3
57	Frequently feel drowsy	0	1	2	3
58	Difficulty making decisions	0	1	2	3
59	Often have blurred vision	0	1	2	3
60	Feel you lack sex drive	0	1	2	3
61	Often have muscle twitching or jerking	0	1	2	3
62	Feel better after eating	0	1	2	3
63	Get sleepy/drowsy after lunch	0	1	2	3

Vitamin B Deficiency

		0	1	2	3
64	Enlarged heart and/or heart failure	0	1	2	3
65	Pulse slow (below 65) or irregular pulse	0	1	2	3
66	Low blood pressure	0	1	2	3
67	Varicose veins (spider veins) and/or hemorrhoids	0	1	2	3
68	Slow reflexes	0	1	2	3
69	Irregular heart beat	0	1	2	3
70	Worry, anxiety, insecurity, or highly emotional state	0	1	2	3
71	Sensitive to noises and/or smells	0	1	2	3
72	Have trouble with concentration (foggy-headed)	0	1	2	3
73	Weak digestion (gas, bloating, indigestion)	0	1	2	3
74	Feel drowsy after eating	0	1	2	3
75	Sore and achy muscles after little exercise	0	1	2	3
76	Constantly fatigued	0	1	2	3
77	Wake up at night to urinate	0	1	2	3
78	Wake up at night and can't get back to sleep	0	1	2	3
79	Back pain when in one position (i.e., in bed at night)	0	1	2	3
80	Headband-like headache (like a tight band around head)	0	1	2	3
81	Itchy skin	0	1	2	3
82	Sensitive to insect bites	0	1	2	3
83	Shortness of breath (can't hold breath very long)	0	1	2	3
84	No stamina (get winded easily)	0	1	2	3
85	Frequently yawn	0	1	2	3
86	Low body temperature	0	1	2	3
87	Muscles feel weak (body feels heavy)	0	1	2	3

Vitamin G Deficiency

88	High blood pressure	0	1	2	3
89	Fast heart rate (pulse)	0	1	2	3
90	Muscles feel tense & tight	0	1	2	3
91	Tic-tac rhythm to heart beat (no rest between heart beats)	0	1	2	3
92	Worry excessively (mind races)	0	1	2	3
93	Always tense can't relax	0	1	2	3
94	Tend to be suspicious by nature	0	1	2	3
95	Moody	0	1	2	3
96	Depressed	0	1	2	3
97	Tend to have cold hands & feet	0	1	2	3
98	Weak digestion (gas, bloating, indigestion)	0	1	2	3
99	Muscles restless always moving	0	1	2	3
100	Body jerks when falling asleep	0	1	2	3
101	Aware of muscle twitching	0	1	2	3
102	Feel tight; not flexible	0	1	2	3
103	Trouble digesting fats (indigestion after eating fatty foods)	0	1	2	3
104	Can hear heartbeat in ears (especially lying in bed at night)	0	1	2	3
105	Cracking at the corners of mouth (cheilosis)	0	1	2	3
106	Friable, easily irritated skin (especially after shaving)	0	1	2	3
107	Red, irritated tongue (sometimes purple color to tongue)	0	1	2	3
108	Irritated mucous membranes (sinus, lungs, rectum, etc.)	0	1	2	3
109	Loss of upper lip (thin upper lip)	0	1	2	3
110	Burning or itching of eyes	0	1	2	3
111	Bloodshot eyes	0	1	2	3
112	Eyes sensitive to light (photophobia)	0	1	2	3
113	See only part of printed words (like looking through a fishbowl)	0	1	2	3

Fatty Acids Deficiency

114	Joint or muscle pain	0	1	2	3
115	Glaucoma	0	1	2	3
116	Autoimmune disease (of any kind)	0	1	2	3
117	Cold-sensitive; always feel cold	0	1	2	3
118	Chronic headaches	0	1	2	3
119	Parasthesias (abnormal sensations in body) or neuralgia	0	1	2	3
120	Muscle cramping	0	1	2	3
121	Abrupt changes in visual acuity	0	1	2	3
122	Popping or cracking in ears or tinnitis	0	1	2	3
123	Problems swallowing	0	1	2	3
124	Depression and/or anxiety	0	1	2	3
125	Learning disabilities (ADD, ADHD, etc.)	0	1	2	3
126	Epilepsy or narcolepsy	0	1	2	3
127	Dry or scaling skin (elbows, knees, forearms, shins)	0	1	2	3
128	Phyrnoderma (roughness of upper arms, thighs, buttocks)	0	1	2	3
129	Dandruff or flaking skin, in general	0	1	2	3
130	Psoriasis or eczema	0	1	2	3
131	Dyspigmentation (aging spots, vitiligo)	0	1	2	3
132	Dry or brittle hair	0	1	2	3
133	Acne	0	1	2	3

High Autonomic

134	High blood pressure	0	1	2	3
135	Fast heart rate (pulse)	0	1	2	3
136	Dilated pupils	0	1	2	3
137	Tend toward dry mouth (may have difficulty swallowing)	0	1	2	3
138	Cold, clammy hands and feet	0	1	2	3
139	Excess muscle tension	0	1	2	3
140	Quick reflexes	0	1	2	3
141	Anxious, mind races, and can't relax	0	1	2	3
142	Excessive sweating	0	1	2	3
143	Lots of energy, but poor stamina or nervous exhaustion	0	1	2	3
144	Tendency toward constipation	0	1	2	3
145	Feel like food sits in stomach; queasiness or nausea	0	1	2	3
146	Tendency toward a strong body odor	0	1	2	3
147	Women: Difficult to become sexually aroused	0	1	2	3
148	Men: Difficulty getting an erection or weak erections	0	1	2	3

Low Autonomic

149	Low blood pressure	0	1	2	3
150	Slow heart rate (pulse)	0	1	2	3
151	Constricted pupils	0	1	2	3
152	Tendency toward increased saliva	0	1	2	3
153	Warm, dry skin (warm hands and feet)	0	1	2	3
154	Family history of diabetes or low thyroid	0	1	2	3
155	Slow reflexes	0	1	2	3
156	Unmotivated or lackadaisical	0	1	2	3
157	Calm, even disposition	0	1	2	3
158	Low energy but good endurance	0	1	2	3
159	Get stiff/achy after being in one position (sleeping/sitting)	0	1	2	3
160	Tendency toward laziness or undisciplined behavior	0	1	2	3
161	Women: Strong sex drive; easily aroused	0	1	2	3
162	Men: Easily achieve strong erections; strong sex drive	0	1	2	3

High Pituitary

163	Increased sex drive	0	1	2	3
164	Splitting headaches	0	1	2	3
165	Failing memory	0	1	2	3
166	Working excessively until exhausted	0	1	2	3
167	Feeling keyed up; unable to relax	0	1	2	3
168	Reduced tolerance for sugar	0	1	2	3

Low Pituitary

169	Reduced or absent sex drive	0	1	2	3
170	Abnormal thirst	0	1	2	3
171	Weight gain around hips or waist	0	1	2	3
172	Tendency toward ulcers or colitis	0	1	2	3
173	Ability to eat sugar without symptoms	0	1	2	3
174	Menstrual disorders (women)	0	1	2	3
175	Lack of menstruation (teenage girls)	0	1	2	3

High Thyroid

176	Hard to gain weight despite large appetite	0	1	2	3
177	Heart palpitations	0	1	2	3
178	Nervous, emotional and/or can't work under pressure	0	1	2	3
179	Insomnia	0	1	2	3
180	Inward trembling	0	1	2	3
181	Night sweats	0	1	2	3
182	Fast pulse at rest	0	1	2	3
183	Intolerant of high temperatures	0	1	2	3
184	Easily flushed	0	1	2	3

Low Thyroid

185	Difficulty losing weight	0	1	2	3
186	Reduced initiative and/or mental sluggishness	0	1	2	3
187	Easily fatigued; sleepy during the day	0	1	2	3
188	Sensitive to cold, poor circulation, cold hands and feet	0	1	2	3
189	Dry or scaly skin	0	1	2	3
190	Ringing in ears or noises in head	0	1	2	3
191	Hearing impaired	0	1	2	3
192	Constipation	0	1	2	3
193	Excessive hair loss and/or coarse hair	0	1	2	3
194	Headache upon waking; wears off during day	0	1	2	3

High Adrenal

195	Elevated blood pressure		1	2	3
196	Headaches	0	1	2	3
197	Hot flashes	0	1	2	3
198	Hair growth on face or body (females)	0	1	2	3
199	Masculine tendencies (females)	0	1	2	3

Low Adrenal

200	Low blood pressure	0	1	2	3
201	Crave salt	0	1	2	3
202	Chronic fatigue or drowsiness	0	1	2	3
203	Afternoon yawning	0	1	2	3
204	Feeling tired upon waking	0	1	2	3
205	Weakness or dizziness	0	1	2	3
206	Weakness after colds or slow recovery	0	1	2	3
207	Poor circulation	0	1	2	3
208	Muscular and nervous exhaustion	0	1	2	3
209	Susceptible to colds, asthma, or bronchitis	0	1	2	3
210	Allergies and/or hives	0	1	2	3
211	Difficulty holding chiropractic adjustments	0	1	2	3
212	Arthritic tendencies	0	1	2	3
213	Nails weak and/or ridged	0	1	2	3
214	Perspire easily	0	1	2	3
215	Slow starter in the morning	0	1	2	3
216	Afternoon headaches	0	1	2	3

Nutritional Deficiency

		0	1	2	3
217	Frequent skin rashes and/or hives	0	1	2	3
218	Muscle cramping of leg or foot when at rest or sleeping	0	1	2	3
219	Fevers easily raised or frequent	0	1	2	3
220	Crave chocolate	0	1	2	3
221	Feet have bad odor	0	1	2	3
222	Frequent hoarseness	0	1	2	3
223	Difficulty swallowing	0	1	2	3
224	Joint stiffness upon arising	0	1	2	3
225	Frequent vomiting	0	1	2	3
226	Tendency to anemia	0	1	2	3
227	Whites of eyes (sclera) blue	0	1	2	3
228	Lump in throat	0	1	2	3
229	Dryness of eyes, mouth, and/or nose	0	1	2	3
230	White spots on fingernails	0	1	2	3
231	Cuts heal slowly and/or scar easily	0	1	2	3
232	Reduced/lost sense of taste and/or smell	0	1	2	3
233	Susceptible to colds, fevers, and/or infections	0	1	2	3
234	Strong light irritates eyes	0	1	2	3
235	Noises in head or ringing in ears	0	1	2	3
236	Burning sensations in mouth	0	1	2	3
237	Numbness in hands and feet	0	1	2	3
238	Intolerant to MSG	0	1	2	3
239	Cannot recall dreams	0	1	2	3
240	Frequent nosebleeds	0	1	2	3
241	Bruise easily	0	1	2	3
242	Muscle cramping; worse with exercise	0	1	2	3

Heart Function

		0	1	2	3
243	Aware of heavy and/or irregular breathing	0	1	2	3
244	Discomfort at high altitude	0	1	2	3
245	"Air hunger"; sigh frequently	0	1	2	3
246	Swollen ankles, worse at night	0	1	2	3
247	Shortness of breath with exertion	0	1	2	3
248	Dull pain in chest or radiating into arm, worse with exertion	0	1	2	3

Female Hormonal

		0	1	2	3
249	Premenstrual tension	0	1	2	3
250	Painful menses (cramping, etc.)	0	1	2	3
251	Menstruation excessive or prolonged	0	1	2	3
252	Painful or tender breasts	0	1	2	3
253	Menstruate too frequently	0	1	2	3
254	Acne, worse at menses	0	1	2	3
255	Depressed feeling before menstruation	0	1	2	3
256	Vaginal discharge	0	1	2	3
257	Menses scanty or missed	0	1	2	3
258	Hysterectomy or ovaries removed	0	1	2	3
259	Menopausal hot flashes	0	1	2	3
260	Depression	0	1	2	3

Male Hormonal

261	Prostate trouble	0	1	2	3
262	Urination difficult or dribbling	0	1	2	3
263	Frequent night urination	0	1	2	3
264	Pain on inside of legs or heels	0	1	2	3
265	Feeling of incomplete bowel movement	0	1	2	3
266	Leg nervousness at night	0	1	2	3
267	Tire easily; avoid activity	0	1	2	3
268	Reduced sex drive	0	1	2	3
269	Depression	0	1	2	3
270	Migrating aches and pains	0	1	2	3

Health Graph

Name: _____ Date ___/___/___ Test #: ___

Organ/System	Total	%T	10%	20%	30%	40%	50%	60%	70%	80%	90%	100%
Digestion Problems	/21											
Liver/Gall Bladder	/48											
Large Intestine	/18											
Allergies	/21											
Immune System	/15											
Blood Sugar Problems	/66											
Vitamin B Deficiency	/72											
Vitamin G Deficiency	/78											
Fatty Acids Deficiency	/60											
High Autonomic	/42											
Low Autonomic	/39											
High Pituitary	/18											
Low Pituitary	/21											
High Thyroid	/27											
Low Thyroid	/30											
High Adrenal	/15											
Low Adrenal	/48											
Nutritional Deficiency	/78											
Heart Function	/18											
Female Hormonal	/36											
Male Hormonal	/30											

	Main Symptoms		Percent Symptoms Improve									
1												
2												
3												
4												
5												

OVERVIEW: _____

_____

_____

Home Tests Form

Name:

Date:				
Pulse (Ideal Range: 50-70 BPM)				
Sitting Blood Pressure (Ideal: 120/80) Ideal Range: 114-130/76-86				
Lying Blood Pressure				
Lying Blood Pressure Change (+/-) Norm: Slight drop in Diastolic				
Standing Blood Pressure				
Standing Blood Pressure Change (+/-) Norm: Increase Systolic 4-10mmHg <4mmHg = Low Adrenal >10mmHg = High Adrenal, High Pituitary or Sympathetic Dominant				
Saliva pH (Norm: 7.2)				
Urine pH (Norm: 6.5)				
Temperature (4-day average) Ideal Range: 97.8-98.2 <97.8 = Low Thyroid, Low Pituitary, Low Adrenal, or Vitamin B Deficiency >98.2 = High Thyroid, High Pituitary, acute or chronic infection				
Zinc Taste Test 1 = No taste = Markedly zinc-deficient 2 = Slight, delayed taste = Zinc-deficient 3 = Distinct taste = Slightly zinc-deficient 4 = Very strong/unpleasant taste = Good				
Oxidation Stress Test +3 = Marked antoxidant need +2 = Definite antioxidant need +1 = Probable antioxidant need 0 = No antioxidant need				
Urine Calcium (Sulkowitch Test) 1 = Clear = Marked calcium deficiency 2 = Slightly cloudy = Calcium deficiency 3 = Moderately cloudy = Normal 4 = Milky = Excess calcium				
Urine Sodium (Koenisburg Test) 18-22 = Normal 24 or greater = Low Adrenal 16 or lower = High Adrenal or Low Adrenal at Stage II exhaustion				

Lab Tests

Name: _____ **Lab Sheet #:** _____

Date:				
Electrolyte Balance				
Magnesium	>2.0			
Potassium	4.0–4.5			
Sodium	135–142			
Chloride	100–106			
Energy				
Glucose	80–95			
Glycated Hemoglobin	<7			
Carbon Dioxide	26-31			
Protein				
BUN	10–16			
Creatinine	.8-1.1			
Uric Acid	(F) 3.0–5.5 (M) 3.5–5.9			
Total Protei n	6.8–7.4			
Albumin	4.0–4.9			
Globulin	2.4–2.8			
Blood Count				
RBC	(F) 3.9–4.5 (M) 4.2–4.9			
HgB	(F) 13.5–14.5 (M) 14.0–15.0			
Hct	(F) 37.0–44.0 (M) 40.0–48.0%			
MCV	82–89.9			
MCH	27.0–31.9%			
WBC	5,000–7,500			
Neutrophils	40–60%			
Lymphocytes	24–44%			
Monocytes	0–7%			
Eosinophiols	0–3%			
Basophils	0–1%			

Lab Tests

Name: _____   **Lab Sheet #:** _____

Date:				
Calcium & Phosphorus				
Calcium	9.4–10.0			
Phosphorous	3.0–4.0			
Ca/P Ratio	~2.4			
Blood Fats				
Cholesterol	150–220			
LDL	120 or less			
HDL	(F) >60 (M) >55			
Triglycerides	70–110			
Thyroid				
T-3 Uptake	27–37%			
T3 RIA (Total T3)	100–230			
T-4 (Thyroxine)	6–12			
T7 (FTI)	same as lab norms			
TSH	2.0-4.4			
Liver & Gall Bladder				
LDH	140–200			
Alkaline Phosphatase	70–100			
SGOT (AST)	10–30			
SGPT (ALT)	10–30			
GGTP	10–30			
Total Bilirubin	0.1-1.2			

Available from The Elements of Health

Product	Description	Price
choosing **HEALTH** Workbook	Think of all of your friends and family who can enjoy better health and wellbeing by *choosing* **HEALTH**	$29.95
choosing **HEALTH** Newsletter	Keep up-to-date with new developments in functional selfcare, new research in the healing arts, and tips on how to use *choosing* **HEALTH**. Monthly. Via e-mail ... FREE Regular mail ... $18.00	FREE / $18.00
choosing **HEALTH** Daily Journal	Helps you to incorporate the elements of health into your daily lifestyle, keeps track of your follow-up self-testing, and gives insight into more fully using the tools from *choosing* **HEALTH**	$15.00
choosing **HEALTH** Video	This video has Dr. Force introducing the concepts and methods from *choosing* **HEALTH**, plus he'll show you how to conduct, chart, and interpret the health graph, home tests, and lab tests.	$19.95
choosing **HEALTH** Software	Automated charting, interpretation, and recommendations. In development.	
Home Test Kit	This is a complete kit for doing the Home Tests covered in *choosing* **HEALTH**. Includes a mercury thermometer, pH paper, and the oxidation stress, Zinc, Calcium, and Sodium tests. If purchased separately, $75.00	$60.00
Thermometer	Mercury thermometers are hard to find anymore and are the only accurate way to take temperatures	$6.00
Ph Paper	The pH range is 5-8. Perfect for checking urine and saliva pH	$6.00
Oxidation Stress Test	Tests for antioxidant need	$12.00
Zinc Taste Test	Comes as liquid and allows many tests	$13.00
Calcium Test	Measures body calcium levels	$13.00
Sodium Test	Essential for measuring adrenal function and the effects	$13.00

The Elements of Health

7500 E. Pinnacle Peak Rd., Suite A-207
Scottsdale AZ 85255
Phone: 480-563-4256
Toll-free: 866-563-4256
Fax: 480-563-4269
Email: info@theelementsofhealth.com
Web: theelementsofhealth.com